TECHNICAL
REPORT

Living Conditions in Anbar Province in June 2008

Keith Crane, Martin C. Libicki, Audra K. Grant, James B. Bruce, Omar Al-Shahery, Alireza Nader, Suzanne Perry

Sponsored by the U.S. Department of Defense

RAND NATIONAL DEFENSE RESEARCH INSTITUTE

The research described in this report was sponsored by the U.S. Department of Defense and conducted in the RAND National Defense Research Institute, a federally funded research and development center sponsored by the Office of the Secretary of Defense, the Joint Staff, the Unified Combatant Commands, the Department of the Navy, the Marine Corps, the defense agencies, and the defense Intelligence Community under Contract W74V8H-06-C-0002.

Library of Congress Cataloging-in-Publication Data

Living conditions in Anbar Province in June 2008 / Keith Crane ... [et al.].
p. cm.
Includes bibliographical references.
ISBN 978-0-8330-4752-6 (pbk. : alk. paper)
1. Anbar (Iraq : Province)—Social conditions. 2. Anbar (Iraq : Province)—Economic conditions. 3. Quality of life—Anbar (Iraq : Province) 4. Social indicators—Anbar (Iraq : Province) 5. Economic indicators—Anbar (Iraq : Province) I. Crane, Keith, 1953–

HN670.A925L58 2009
304.6'1095674—dc22

2009029223

Published 2009 by the RAND Corporation
1776 Main Street, P.O. Box 2138, Santa Monica, CA 90407-2138
1200 South Hayes Street, Arlington, VA 22202-5050
4570 Fifth Avenue, Suite 600, Pittsburgh, PA 15213-2665
RAND URL: http://www.rand.org/
To order RAND documents or to obtain additional information, contact
Distribution Services: Telephone: (310) 451-7002;
Fax: (310) 451-6915; Email: order@rand.org

Preface

The local population is the center of gravity in counterinsurgency. The first step toward winning the population is to understand it. To this end, the RAND Corporation, in spring 2008, conducted a survey of Iraq's Anbar Province by putting a detailed set of questions to 1,200 randomly selected households. The survey was designed to collect a wide variety of data—ranging from demographics and housing to employment and living standards—about Anbari households and citizens. This report summarizes the key results of the survey; a companion report covering the results of a second survey to be conducted in June 2009 will be published in fall 2009.

Al-Anbar has been surveyed before, notably in 2004, when the Iraqi government, with cooperation from the United Nations Development Programme (UNDP) and Fafo-AIS, carried out a countrywide survey, reporting results in 2005 on a province-by-province basis. Since 2004, a great deal has transpired in Iraq, notably in al-Anbar. Hence, a new survey was needed to understand current conditions in the province, including the effects of war on the people.

This research was sponsored by the U.S. Department of Defense and conducted within the Intelligence Policy Center of the RAND National Defense Research Institute, a federally funded research and development center sponsored by the Office of the Secretary of Defense, the Joint Staff, the Unified Combatant Commands, the Department of the Navy, the Marine Corps, the defense agencies, and the defense Intelligence Community.

For more information on RAND's Intelligence Policy Center, contact the Director, John Parachini. He can be reached by email at John_Parachini@rand.org; by phone at 703-413-1100, extension 5579; or by mail at the RAND Corporation, 1200 South Hayes Street, Arlington, Virginia 22202-5050. More information about RAND is available at www.rand.org.

Contents

Figures

Tables

Summary

In Iraq's Anbar Province, the local population is, as is typical in any counterinsurgency campaign, the center of gravity. For the forces of order to appeal to the people, security forces need not only to engage in combat but also to understand the people—their concerns, their hopes, their grievances, and how they think and live. To gain a better understanding of how Anbaris live, the RAND Corporation conducted a survey of living conditions in the province. Face-to-face interviews were conducted with a random sample of 1,200 heads of Anbari households (here, defined as a family and other related individuals normally living in one housing unit) between May 28 and June 10, 2008. Interviews were conducted by local Anbaris, who were trained over four days by instructors who had attended a separate training course held outside Iraq and conducted by RAND and subcontractor staff. While one might expect respondents to react with some hesitancy toward a survey asking questions about their daily lives, the response rate averaged 71 percent, a figure on par with response rates for similar surveys in other Middle Eastern countries. The survey produced a wealth of data, which are available to researchers upon request from RAND. The survey's main findings are summarized below.

Demographics

Violence has left its mark on Anbaris: Many households are headed by widows. Of the 1,200 households surveyed in 2008, females headed 171, or 14 percent—a 4-percent increase over the 2004 figure reported by the Iraqi government.[1] In light of the importance that Anbaris place on minimizing contact between women and men outside their families, when entering homes, both Iraqi security forces and U.S. forces need to be aware that the home may be headed by a female and must offer her due respect and courtesy.

Losing a father is common: Approximately 20 percent of 8-year-olds and almost 40 percent of 20-year-olds have suffered such a loss. The coming of age of large numbers of fatherless young men in a society that puts a premium on revenge is a highly worrisome development for a region emerging from civil war.

[1] Throughout this report, 2004 data are from Ministry of Planning and Development Cooperation, *Iraq Living Conditions Survey 2004*, Vol. II: *Analytical Report*, Baghdad: Central Organization for Statistics and Information Technology, Ministry of Planning and Development Cooperation, 2005, unless otherwise noted.

Employment

No men over age 23—and no females of any age—are unemployed. Most employment occurs in small, private enterprises. Women are rarely in the labor force (i.e., they are rarely working or actively looking for work), but when they are, their wages are comparable to what men earn. **Because the survey shows that young people eventually find work, Iraqi government and U.S. assistance programs should be focused on training rather than on employment generation. This focus will help raise the potential lifetime earnings of young people by providing them with better skills.** Construction, retail and wholesale trade, and transport are the major employment sectors.

Income and Standards of Living

As a province, al-Anbar is recovering economically. Households have more income—and many more consumer durables—than they had four years ago. Nevertheless, most households depend on several sources of income; salaried (mainly government) jobs are uncommon. Anbaris earn most of their income from work of one sort or another. With the great exception of food rations, which almost everyone receives, only a small percentage of income arises from transfers. More money comes from rentals and property sales, but the percentage of income arising from the sale of large assets (e.g., houses) has declined sharply from 2007 levels—a sign that economic distress is dissipating. Higher levels of education are not correlated with higher incomes. However, they *are* associated with a greater likelihood of holding a salaried job.

Ownership of ovens, stoves, televisions, and satellite receivers is universal. Half of all families even have cars. **Every household has access to a cell phone, and all report their service is reliable.** Internet access is common, but almost everyone must visit a cybercafé to use the Internet. Anbaris do continue to experience difficulty in obtaining big-ticket items. Savings, whether held in banks or in gold, are modest. Faced with unexpected expenses, such as weddings or funerals, the typical household needs help.

Education

The population in al-Anbar is for the most part a literate one. Both urban and rural inhabitants have similar rates of literacy; there is also little variation by gender. Virtually all children under the age of 16 are reported to be receiving education. However, a substantial share of Anbaris over the age of 55 received little or no education. Reflecting nationwide patterns of school attendance, about as many Anbaris in the general population are currently enrolled in some type of educational institution as are not. When young Anbaris are not literate, it is usually the result of a lack of access to schools due to their destruction during the war, a lack of transportation, and concerns that it is still too dangerous to attend.

Health

According to respondents, the four greatest problems with health care in al-Anbar are (1) the fact that a large number of health care professionals have left Iraq, (2) the lack of supplies and equipment, (3) the limited range of health services available nearby, and (4) unsanitary facilities.

When Anbaris become ill, 40 percent go to licensed physicians. A smaller portion go to nurses, but a considerable percentage uses unlicensed pharmacists (drugs are easily dispensed in al-Anbar). Nongovernmental and international organizations provide a large part of the population with the kind of services they used to get from government-run health care centers. Health care remains relatively inexpensive: Depending on the services sought, only 20–40 percent of all households report that affordability is a problem. Yet, Anbaris find it difficult to get appointments with professionals, a problem largely due to the fact that so many professionals have fled the province.

Housing and Public Infrastructure

Crowded living conditions, limited access to water, and sporadic supplies of electric power remain problems in al-Anbar. In the average household—with its seven or eight people—members sleep in one of three bedrooms. Electric power supply remains erratic, with over half of all households experiencing daily outages; in a quarter of all households, the power is off more often than on. All households supplement power from the grid with power from diesel-powered generators, which are shared with neighbors, operated by a neighborhood cooperative, or run by a private local company. Water supply is also unreliable. **However, survey respondents report that access to health care, electricity, and water is improving, although access levels are still unsatisfactory to much of the population.**

Anbaris have better access to mosques than to police stations. Ninety percent of the population can get to a mosque within 15 minutes. Less than 5 percent can get to a police station that quickly.

The Effects of War

In light of the levels of violence in al-Anbar since 2003, it is unsurprising that nearly all respondents report having been affected by war. **Nearly half of households say that a household member has been killed as a result of the conflict.** Many report that household members have disappeared, been detained, or been arrested. Exposure to crime is another byproduct of the violent conflict.

Eighteen percent of the households surveyed reported that at least one member had relocated since 2003. Violence was the main reason cited for leaving. Roughly half (59 percent) of survey respondents said that the household member who left migrated to Syria; the other members went to Jordan (12 percent), Egypt (8 percent), Sweden (6 percent), and elsewhere (15 percent).

Agriculture

Surprisingly, the role of agriculture was similar in urban and rural households. The divide between urban and rural cultures in al-Anbar is blurred; nearly everyone lives near the Euphrates and in relatively densely populated areas. **Forty percent of all households—urban and rural alike—own agricultural land; roughly the same percentage farm it, although farming is typically a secondary source of income and food.** Rural and urban households are equally as likely to own livestock. As levels of violence fell and economic activity increased between 2007 and 2008, holdings of livestock rose.

Acknowledgments

The RAND research team did not conduct the survey or write this report alone. We have a great many people to thank for their assistance in helping to bring this report to fruition. We are grateful to Jon Pederson and Kristen Dalen of Fafo for their advice and for providing the original questionnaires and training manuals used during the 2004 survey in both English and Arabic. Because we were able to ask so many questions originally asked during the 2004 survey, we were able to make comparisons over time that otherwise would have been impossible. Professor Frank Gunter of Lehigh University generously provided his insights on the Iraqi economy and society, helping us to better tailor our revisions to the 2004 questionnaire. We would also like to thank L. Andrew Jones, Research Protections Manager, Department of the Navy, Human Research Protections Program, Office of Naval Research, and Charles Ries, formerly of the U.S. Mission Baghdad, for their assistance in getting permission to conduct this survey. Scott Carroll and Charles Ries of RAND provided two very helpful reviews of the manuscript. At RAND, we received valuable statistical support from Bonnie Ghosh Dastidar, Louis T. Mariano, Mathias Schonlau, Christine E. Peterson, and Annie Zhou. We thank Ghassan Schbley and Natasha Hall for assisting with the research effort. We are grateful to Kathi Webb for her valuable comments. We also thank Joya Laha for her administrative support.

Abbreviations

AQI	al-Qaeda in Iraq
CERP	Commander's Emergency Response Program
COSIT	Central Office for Statistics and Information Technology
NGO	nongovernmental organization
PC	personal computer
PSU	primary sampling unit
SP	sampling point
UNDP	United Nations Development Programme

CHAPTER ONE

Introduction and Methodology

Iraq's Anbar Province in 2008 was a very different place than it was in 2006. Then, the likely outcome of the struggle between al-Qaeda in Iraq (AQI) on the one hand and Coalition forces, the local population, and the governing institutions of the province on the other was anything but clear. Since that period, the level of violence has dropped dramatically. Life is becoming more normal, and politics has begun to replace violence as a way to settle disputes.[1]

However, conditions in al-Anbar could cease to improve or could even deteriorate. AQI could recover enough strength to renew attacks, especially if it has sleeper cells in place waiting for propitious opportunities. The relationship between the mostly Sunni province and the Shia-dominated central government is tense. Recovery from years of violence is by no means complete.

In al-Anbar, the local population is, as in any counterinsurgency campaign, the center of gravity. The first step toward winning the population is to understand it. For the forces of order to appeal to the people, security forces need to understand not just politics but also how the people live.

One means of obtaining such understanding is to survey the local population concerning its living conditions. To this end, during the end of May and early June 2008, RAND conducted a survey of al-Anbar. The survey involved putting a detailed set of questions to the heads of 1,200 randomly selected households. It was designed to collect a wide variety of data—ranging from demographics and housing to employment and living standards—about Anbari households and citizens.

A primary purpose of the project was to identify key areas on which to focus assistance or Iraqi government funds in al-Anbar so as to better address shortfalls in public services. To this end, the survey asked households about their access to electric power, water, sewage services, health care, and education. The survey also asked detailed questions about educational qualifications, employment, and incomes so as to better inform decisions about investments in education and economic development.

Another major purpose of the survey was to collect information on the effects of war. We asked questions about household-member deaths, injuries, and incarcerations, and about whether members of the household had fled the province. We also asked households whether any members had moved to al-Anbar from elsewhere in Iraq. The data received provide some information on displacement, which will help estimate the numbers of internally displaced people and refugees.

---

[1] See, for example, Sudarsan Raghavan, "A New Breed Grabs Reins in Anbar," *Washington Post*, October 22, 2008.

Al-Anbar has been surveyed before, notably in 2004, when the Iraqi government, with cooperation from the United Nations Development Programme (UNDP) and Fafo-AIS, a Norwegian nonprofit research group, carried out a countrywide survey, reporting results in 2005 on a province-by-province basis. Since 2004, a great deal has transpired in Iraq, notably in al-Anbar. Hence, a new survey was needed to understand current conditions in the province, including the effects of war on the people.

Methodology

The survey consisted of face-to-face interviews with the heads of 1,200 Anbari households (here, defined as a family and other related individuals normally living in one housing unit) between May 28 and June 10, 2008. The interviews averaged a little over two hours each. The survey was conducted by an Iraqi survey firm, a subsidiary of a larger firm, to which RAND subcontracted the survey work. The company employed 31 interviewers, 15 male and 16 female, for this survey. Male and female interviewers were paired with one another to reassure the interviewees and to elicit more-open responses from female heads of household. Interviewers were trained over four days by supervisors who had completed a separate two-day training session delivered by RAND and subcontractor staff.

Survey Instrument

The survey asked the heads of household to answer retrospective questions as well as questions about living conditions in May–June 2008. The survey questionnaire was based on the one used during the Iraqi government's 2004 survey, which was conducted by the Central Organization for Statistics and Information Technology (COSIT) and, as previously noted, supported by UNDP and Fafo. Fafo managed that earlier survey, writing the questionnaire, supervising translation, selecting the sample, conducting pretests, and conducting the final analysis.[2] Although the RAND questionnaire generally replicated the nationwide 2004 survey, some items were altered in order to capture different aspects of the original measures. However, because most questions were identical, we were able to compare the findings from the 2008 survey with those from the 2004 survey.[3]

The 2008 survey included questions on family structure, employment patterns, consumption, income levels, and access to public services. Retrospective questions asked about living conditions in prior periods, usually 12 months prior to the survey. In a number of instances (e.g., in the cases of employment status and income), we posed the same question twice, asking once about the current period and once about a year earlier.

In addition to seeking to understand living conditions among the citizens of once-restive al-Anbar, we also sought to establish benchmarks for developing quantifiable measures of change in quality of life over time. Findings from this survey should be helpful for assess-

[2] Fafo kindly provided us with the original survey instrument in both English and Arabic. COSIT surveyed a random sample of 21,668 Iraqi households. Most households were surveyed during April and May 2004, but surveys in Erbil and Dahuk were conducted in August 2004.

[3] A number of the 2004 survey's questions on agriculture, maternal health, and child health were not included in the 2008 survey. Other questions were shortened or slightly modified. The 2008 survey instrument is available upon request from James Bruce at james_bruce@rand.org.

ing the effectiveness of past assistance programs and targeting future programs for maximum effectiveness. The results also shed light on the relationship between stability and the prospects for improvement in living conditions.

Multistage Sampling Framework

Households were randomly selected on the basis of a stratified cluster sample. The selection methodology was designed to yield statistically valid results that may be generalized to the entire population of al-Anbar. RAND first stratified al-Anbar into four regions or strata: Ramadi, Fallujah, other urban areas, and rural areas. The number of sampling points (SPs) used in each stratum was determined according to population estimates for that stratum. The population estimates were for mid-2005 and were generated by COSIT in August 2005. Although COSIT's detailed methodology for estimating Iraq's population has not been made publicly available, the U.S. Census Bureau has been providing methodological assistance to COSIT for census studies and estimates since 2003. COSIT estimates of local populations are used by the Multi-National Force–Iraq and the Government of Iraq for reconstruction efforts, elections, and conducting policy referenda. The estimates are available at the province and district levels for 15 of Iraq's Arab-majority provinces, but not for the Kurdish region (the Kurds operate their own statistical services separately from COSIT). The estimates are based in part on the 1997 Iraqi census.

The second sampling stage included the selection of districts, towns, and villages within the four strata. This phase determined the primary sampling units (PSUs). The PSUs were randomly selected based on probabilities proportionate to the estimated population of cities or districts within the al-Anbar governorate. Al-Anbar consists of seven cities or districts, all of which were included in this sample.

In the third stage, we selected SPs within the PSUs. The villages within assigned rural PSUs, and the streets within assigned urban PSUs, were defined as SPs. These SPs were selected randomly if a list of all possible urban sampling points (i.e., streets) or rural sampling points (i.e., villages) existed. If not, the area was divided into numbered grids, and the selection was made randomly from these official or informal grid maps. The grid area was small enough to locate as SPs either one or a few villages in rural areas or one or a few streets in urban areas. We selected 173 SPs or geographically clustered areas across the seven districts. These clusters were allocated according to probabilities proportionate to the population of the district.

The fourth stage involved selecting households within the SPs. To control costs, interviewers were asked to interview several households in each SP. However, to minimize the loss of information that might result from interviewing too many households in one SP, we limited the number of households in each cluster to seven. We arrived at this limit by calculating the loss of information that might result from the households in one cluster being more homogeneous vis-à-vis one another than was reflective of al-Anbar as a whole.[4] The selection of households within villages, along streets, or within residential compounds (known as *sokaks*) was accomplished according to the random route-walking principles described below:

[4] Households from a single sampling point may display more similarities with each other than they do with the rest of the households in the province. For example, responses from households in a Chicago neighborhood may be display greater similarity with one another than with responses from a neighborhood in Decatur, Ill.

- The starting point in urban areas was the first household on the left side of the street or sokak. After that, every third household on the route was contacted (yielding a pattern of the first, fourth, seventh, and tenth households being contacted).
- The starting point in rural areas was a central point, such as a mosque, school, or other public building. Facing the building, the walking route proceeded along the left side, starting at the first household on the left side of the street. After that, every third household on the route was contacted (yielding a pattern of the first, fourth, seventh, and tenth households being contacted).

The survey included 173 clusters, 90 of which came from urban areas and 83 of which came from rural areas. This generated a breakdown of 626 urban households and 574 rural households. Fallujah and Ramadi encompassed both urban and rural households.

We interviewed heads of household only. If the head of household refused to be interviewed, or if the interview could not be completed after three callbacks, the interviewer selected another household along the route within the same SP.

Approval for the survey was obtained from the Government of Iraq. The project was also approved by RAND's Human Subject Protection Committee and by the U.S. Department of the Navy's human subject protection procedure.

Factors Influencing the Environment

The survey team contacted a total of 1,692 households, of which 492 refused and 1,200 completed the survey. In other words, the response rate was 71 percent, which is considered robust for most populations. Refusals were distributed across the 173 SPs; none of the SPs exhibited unusual concentrations of refusals. Most households that refused to participate did so outright at the door. We attribute these refusals to concerns about safety. The refusal rate of 29 percent is consistent with the average response rates among populations in the Middle East for surveys of this sort. Because households that refused were replaced with households from the same cluster, the refusals should not have skewed the survey results. The margin of error for the survey was 2.8 percent.

CHAPTER TWO

Demographics

Family Size

Anbari households are large because families have many children.[1] Children tend to leave the household in their early 20s, if they can afford to do so.[2] According to survey results, many such children in al-Anbar cannot do so; therefore, several hundred of the 1,200 surveyed households in the province contain what may be considered secondary families (i.e., children who have married and even had children of their own but have not established a separate household). All the elderly captured in this survey lived with their children. Traditions of caring for parents, limited incomes, and concerns about safety may account for this pattern of secondary families.

Figure 2.1 shows the distribution of households by size; note that there are no households with fewer than three members. The traditional model found in developing-country settings—that larger households predominate in rural areas and smaller households predominate in urban areas—does not appear to hold true in al-Anbar. This may be due to two factors: On the one hand, al-Anbar's cities are not particularly large; on the other hand, the province's rural population densities are not that high (because almost everyone lives close to the Euphrates).

Distribution by Age

In the 2004 survey of Iraq as a whole, the size of the 10-to-14-year-old cohort reached a plateau, with subsequent cohorts (i.e., 5-to-9-year-olds and 0-to-4-year-olds) being only slightly larger;[3] in 2004, 43 percent of the population of Iraq was under age 15. In Table 2.1, which shows the distribution of al-Anbar's population by age, the 15-to-19-year-old cohort (which

---

1 Iraqi households, in general, are large by U.S. standards. The Iraqi government found an average of 6.4 people per household. Al-Anbar, with 8.0 people per household, stood out as having the second-highest household size (second only to Muthanna, with 8.2 people per household). See Ministry of Planning and Development Cooperation, *Iraq Living Conditions Survey 2004*, Vol. II: *Analytical Report*, Baghdad: Central Organization for Statistics and Information Technology, Ministry of Planning and Development Cooperation, 2005.

2 Iraq's social structure is influenced by the dearth of nursing homes and the stigma of sending parents to such facilities. Most families therefore plan for at least one child (almost always male) to remain within their household, primarily to care for parents as they age. After the parents die, that person tends to buy the shares in the house inherited by the other siblings and stay in the home.

3 Throughout this report, 2004 data are from Ministry of Planning and Development Cooperation, 2005, unless otherwise noted.

Figure 2.1
Distribution of 1,200 Households, by Number of Household Members

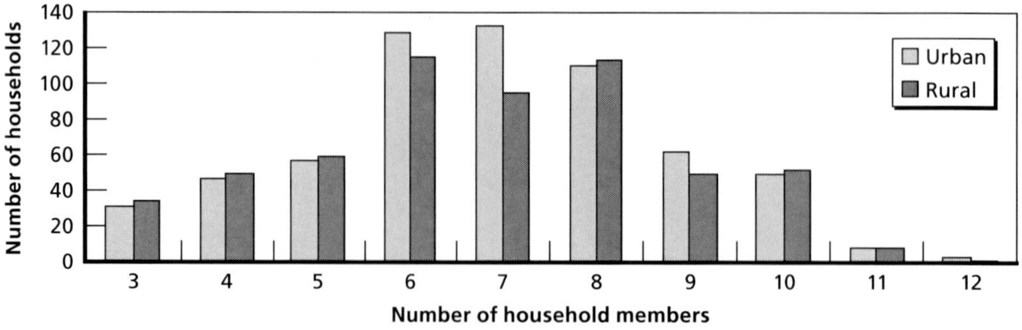

Number of Household Members	Urban	Rural
3	31	34
4	47	49
5	57	59
6	128	115
7	132	95
8	110	113
9	62	49
10	49	52
11	7	7
12	3	1
Total	626	574
Mean	6.9	6.8

RAND *TR715-2.1*

Table 2.1
Distribution of al-Anbar's Population, by Age

Age (years)	Male	Female	Male-to-Female Ratio
≥65	10	5	2.00
60–64	23	6	3.83
55–59	174	96	1.81
50–54	67	158	0.42
45–49	197	218	0.90
40–44	179	241	0.74
35–39	143	129	1.11
30–34	196	116	1.69
25–29	497	339	1.47
20–24	569	438	1.30
15–19	750	368	2.04
10–14	731	432	1.69
5–9	693	447	1.55
≤4	599	380	1.58

mostly overlaps the 10-to-14-year-old cohort of four years earlier) is the largest, with the size of successively younger cohorts roughly the same (see below for an explanation of why there are so few 0-year-olds). In 2008, only 40 percent of the population of al-Anbar was under age 15.[4] The total fertility rate (i.e., the number of children a woman can expect to bear over her lifetime) has fallen in al-Anbar.

Distribution by Sex

One cannot help but notice that there are disproportionately few young women in the sample: 2,520 females under 35 compared with 4,035 males under 35. One would expect an almost equal number of females and males. It is not clear why the anomaly exists. China has a skewed male-to-female ratio (although its ratio of just under 1.2 is lower than al-Anbar's 1.5) among children, but this may be explained by the fact that some families in China, under pressure from the one-child policy, are known to practice selective abortion. In Iraq, there is no such pressure and no indication of such a practice. The most plausible explanation is that many families in al-Anbar did not want to tell interviewers about all their female children. Were we to assume that 1,500 females went unreported by the households surveyed, the average reported household size of 6.8 members is understated: The true number would be closer to 8.1 members, a total closer to the 8.0 members recorded for al-Anbar during the 2004 survey. Hiding females does not appear to be a particularly urban or rural phenomenon.[5] Rural and urban male-to-female ratios are similar, as shown in Figure 2.2.

A similar truncation is visible at the upper end of the age spectrum. Only 28 individuals older than age 60 years were recorded. If al-Anbar's demographics in 2008 were similar to Iraq's demographics in 2004 as estimated in the 2004 survey—which recorded that 4.9 percent of the population was age 60 years or more—we would be seeing far more elderly in the sample. These people may indeed exist in the surveyed households; respondents may have lied about their age or, in some instances, may not have known their true age.

Of the 1,200 households, females head 171, or 14 percent. This 4-percent increase over the 2004 figure may reflect of the effects of the ongoing conflict. Every woman who heads a household is a widow and has children. We found the share of households headed by widows to be strikingly large, and we are almost certain that this is a consequence of the conflict in al-Anbar (both between U.S. forces and Anbaris and between Anbaris and such groups as AQI).

The large proportion of households headed by women in al-Anbar underlines the importance of adapting techniques for entering homes to the realities of the local population. In light of the importance that Anbaris place on minimizing contact between women and men outside their families, when entering homes, both Iraqi security forces

---

[4] Although the 0-to-4-year-old cohort looks substantially smaller than the 5-to-9-year-old cohort, this is entirely due to the size of the 0-year-old cohort, which is half that of the 1-year-old cohort. Absent any good reason to believe that the birthrate dropped by half in 2008 (up to the time of the survey), the best explanation is that most babies born in late 2007 were classified as 1-year-olds even though they had yet to hit their first birthday. We counted these babies in making this generalization.

[5] Discussions with Iraqi survey managers on the issue of "missing females" revealed that it is not at all unusual for households in conflict-ridden societies to attempt to protect female family members by refusing to disclose their existence. The fear is that females might subsequently be exposed to attack.

Figure 2.2
Male-to-Female Ratio, by Age Cohort and Region

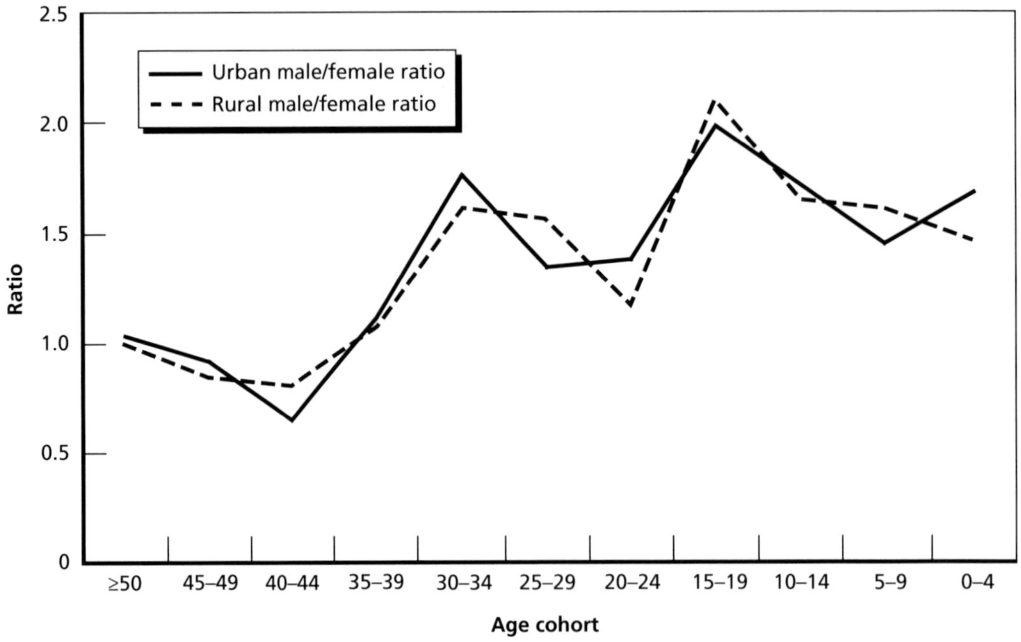

RAND *TR715-2.2*

and U.S. forces need to be aware that the home may be headed by a female and must offer her due respect and courtesy.

The age of the household head is noted in Figure 2.3. Apart from the fact that people in their early 20s do not form households very often (the youngest household-heading female is 33), the distribution is unremarkable (the paucity of men ages 50–54 may be an artifact of how people describe their ages).

Extended Families and Households

Of the 1,200 households surveyed, 862 (over 70 percent) are made of up of only one or more adults plus their unmarried children. The other 30 percent of households contain members who are not part of the nuclear family. Figure 2.4 shows how many such members live in each such household.

Children

Almost half of the households have at least one child under age six. Figure 2.5 enumerates the number of households by the age of their youngest members. Note that every single household has at least one member who is younger than age 26.

Child spacing is fairly close in al-Anbar, and the large families are a consequence of frequent childbirth. Figure 2.6 measures the spacing between childbirths.

If the roughly one-third of girls who are missing come from households that reported their other children, then the calculated birth spacing is even tighter than shown in Figure 2.6.

Figure 2.3
Number of Household Heads, by Age and Sex

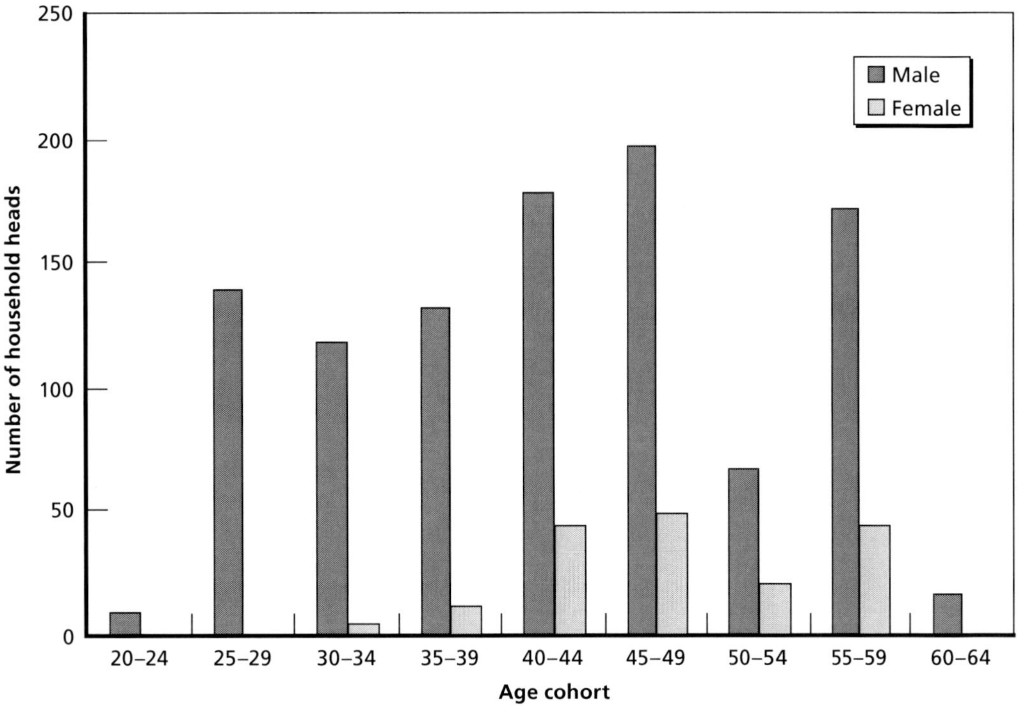

RAND *TR715-2.3*

Figure 2.4
Number of Households with Members Who Are Not Part of the Immediate Family

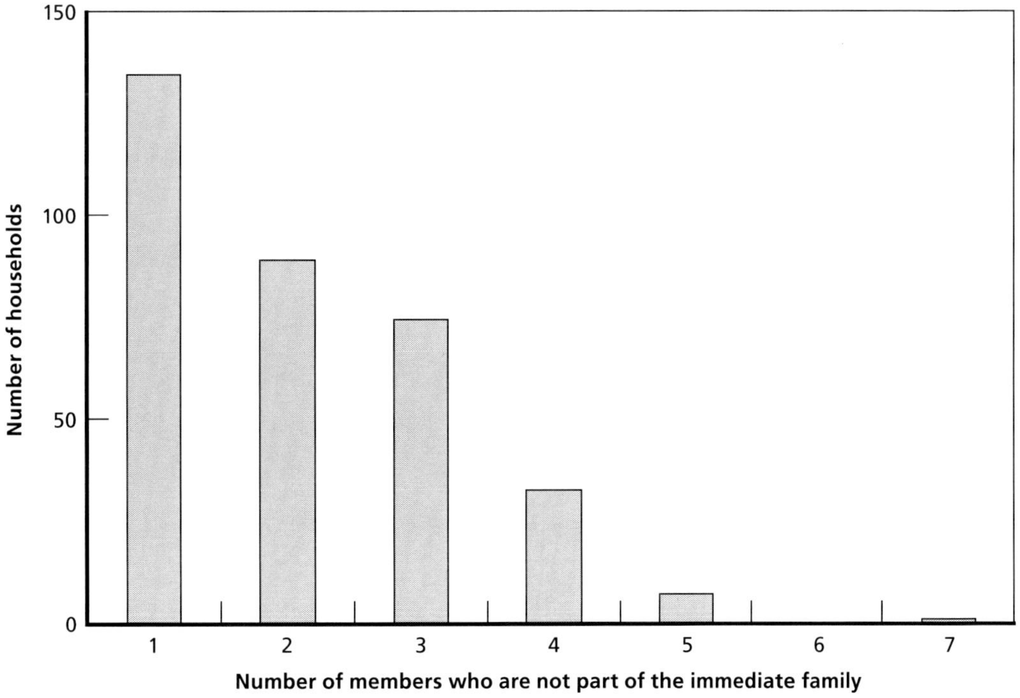

RAND *TR715-2.4*

Figure 2.5
Number of Households, by the Age of the Youngest Member

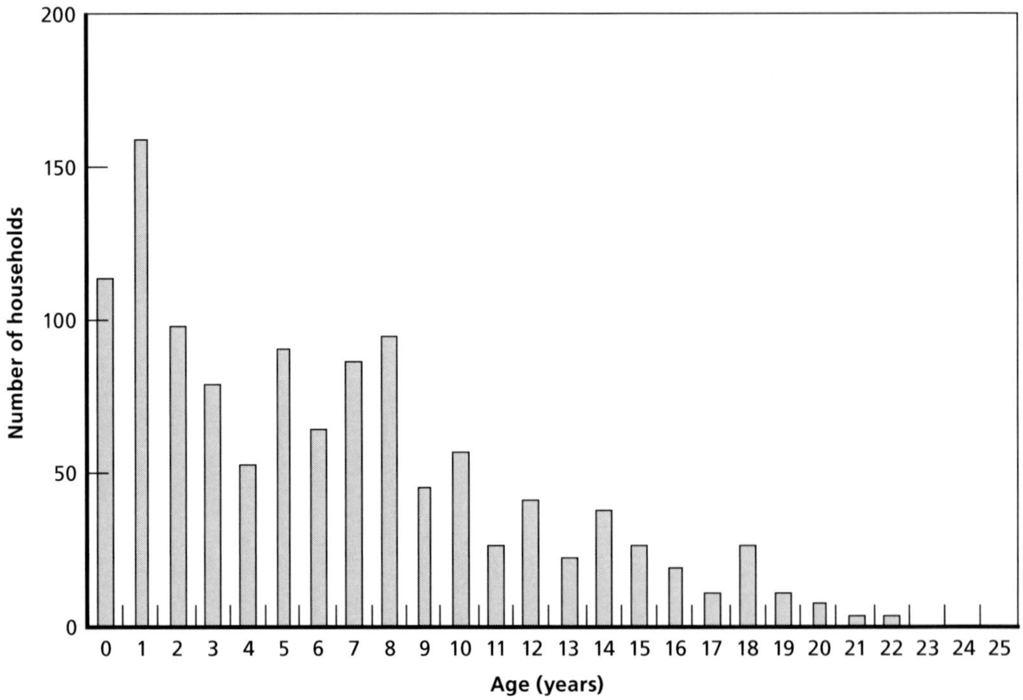

RAND *TR715-2.5*

Figure 2.6
Number of Children, by the Age Difference Between the Child and the Next-Oldest Sibling

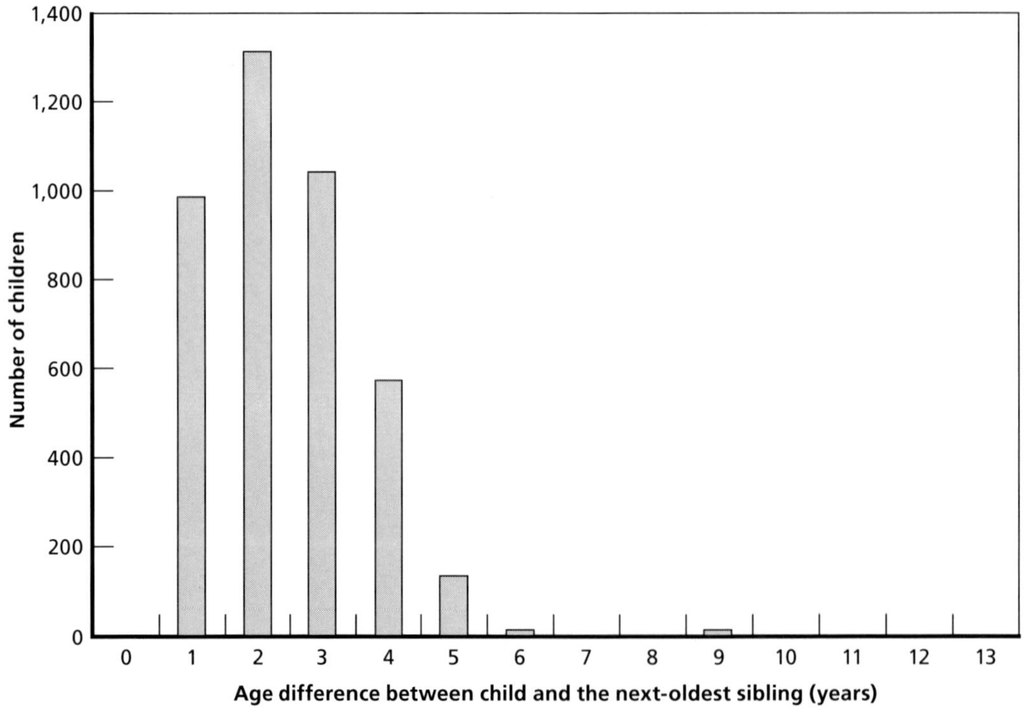

RAND *TR715-2.6*

The missing females may explain why there are only two cases of children being the same age. Twinning normally occurs in roughly one out of every 80 births, a figure that does not count very-closely-spaced siblings.

In a region marked by war, one would expect to see a high number of children who are missing one or both parents. Figure 2.7 displays the percentage of children in each age group who have (1) both parents living, (2) only their mother living, (3) only their father living, or (4) no parents living. The mother of every child age 15 or under is alive. Conversely, by the time a child reaches age eight, his or her chances of losing a father are 20 percent; by age 18, they are almost 40 percent. According to the 2004 survey, fatherless children account for 1 percent of the total; motherless children, 3 percent.

The share of fatherless Anbari children found in this survey is striking, especially compared with the results of the 2004 survey. A large part of this generation of Anbari children, especially teenagers, is coming of age without a father. The coming of age of large numbers of fatherless young men in a society that puts a premium on revenge is a highly worrisome development for a region emerging from civil war.

Marriage

As children grow up, they are wont to marry. Figure 2.7 records the age at marriage of both males and females. The peak marriage age is 24 among females and 25 among males—the relatively late age of marriage for young women is somewhat surprising and may be a consequence of relatively high levels of education in al-Anbar. What is more interesting, at least from

Figure 2.7
Percentage of Children with Living Parents, by the Child's Age

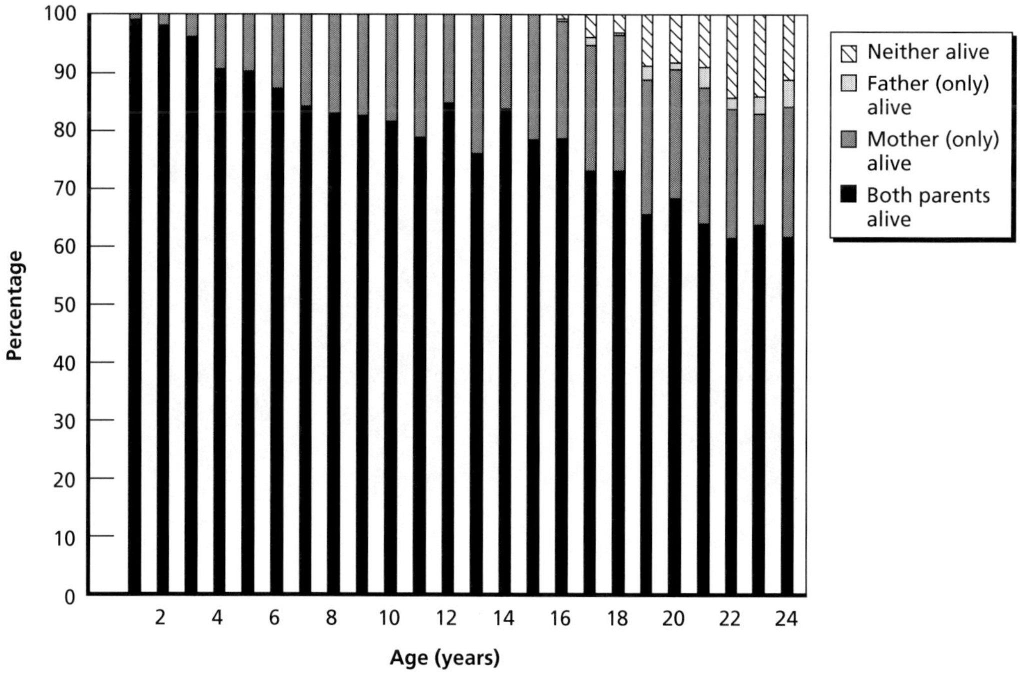

RAND *TR715-2.7*

the U.S. perspective, is the relatively brief age window within which marriage takes place. As shown in Figure 2.8, no man in the sample married after age 32; no woman after age 29. No man married before age 20; no woman married before age 17.

On average, as per Figure 2.9, the male head of household is 3.7 years older than his spouse.

Figures 2.10 and 2.11 show the marriage status of men and women, respectively. First, we note that, although respondents were asked about divorce and separation, no one reported being either divorced or separated. Second, we note that everyone who lives long enough (i.e., to age 37 if male, age 32 if female) eventually gets married. Third, no male under age 60 is a widower.

Figure 2.12 shows the percentage of women in each cohort who are widows, comparing the results from the 2008 survey with those of the 2004 survey. Widowhood is now much more prevalent in al-Anbar.

Figure 2.8
Age of Males and Females at Marriage

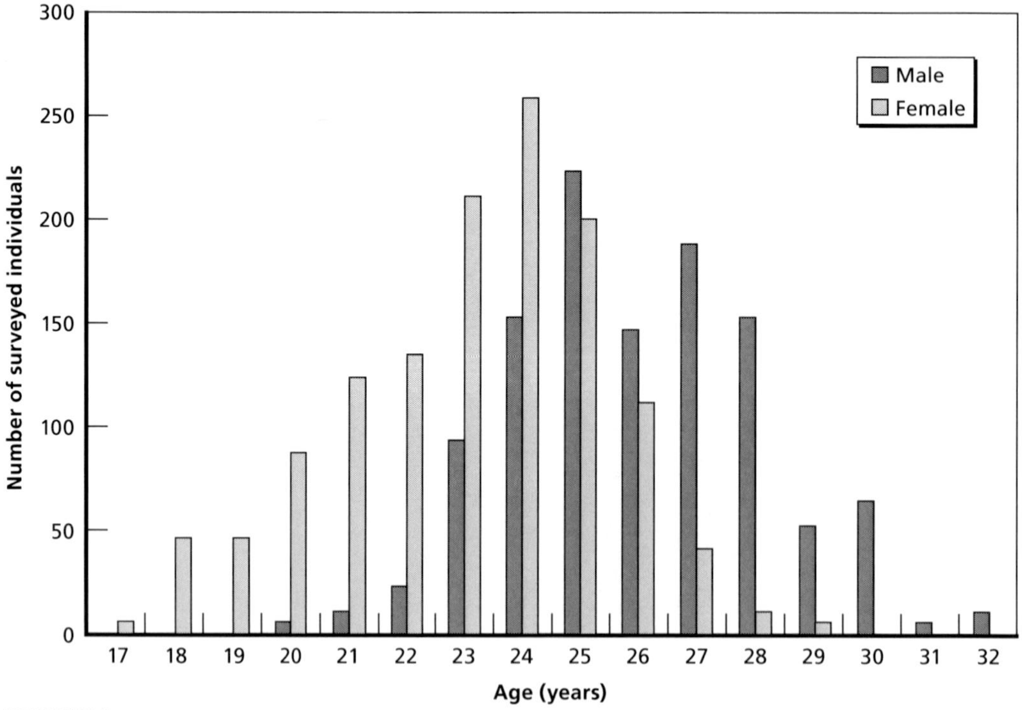

RAND *TR715-2.8*

Figure 2.9
Number of Male-Headed Households, by the Age Difference Between the Husband and the Wife

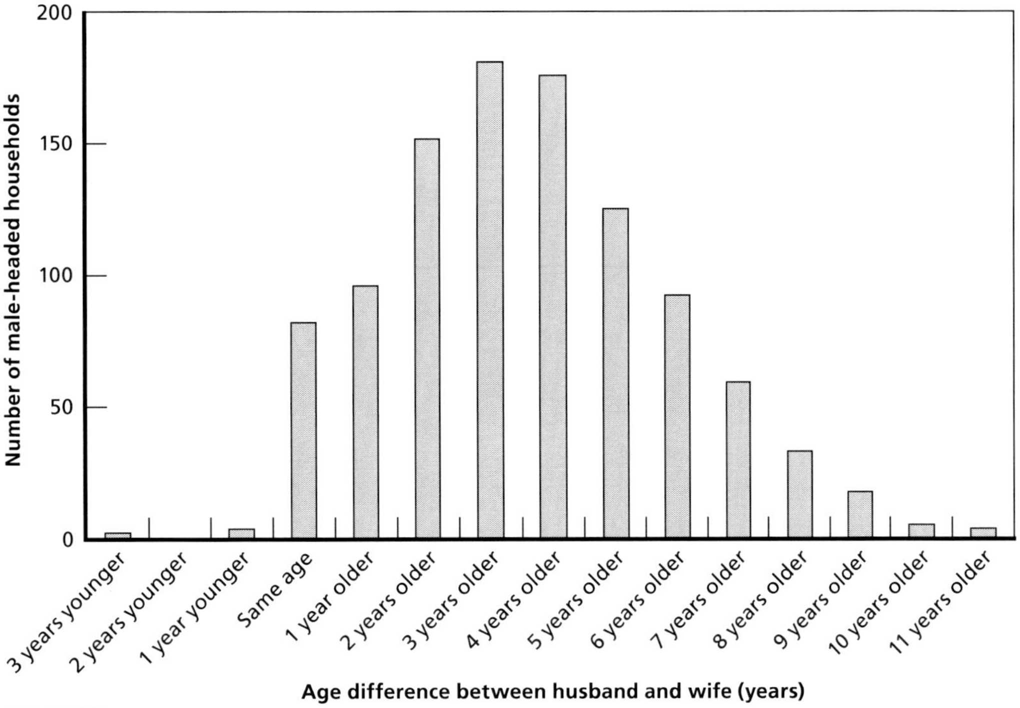

RAND *TR715-2.9*

Figure 2.10
Marital Status of Men, by Age

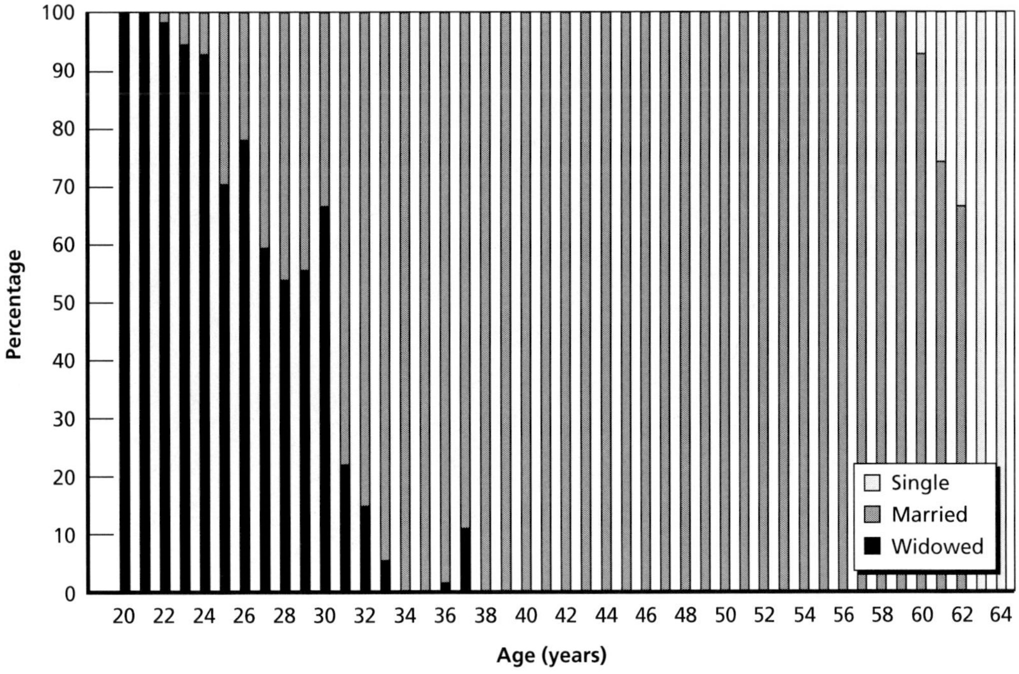

RAND *TR715-2.10*

Figure 2.11
Marital Status of Women, by Age

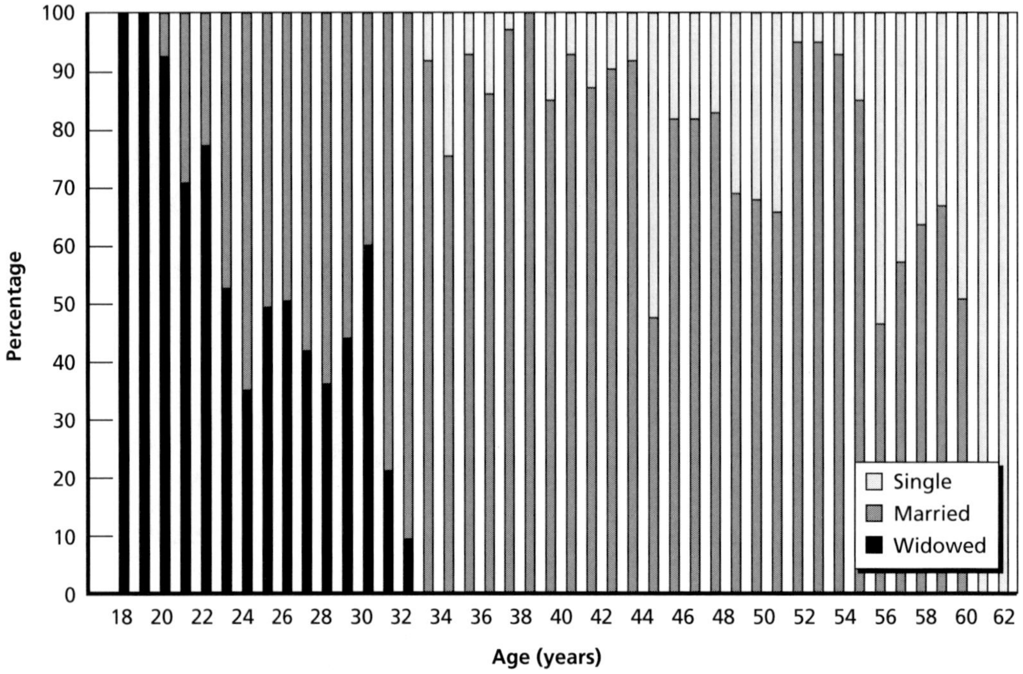

RAND *TR715-2.11*

Figure 2.12
Percentage of Women Who Are Widows, by Age Cohort

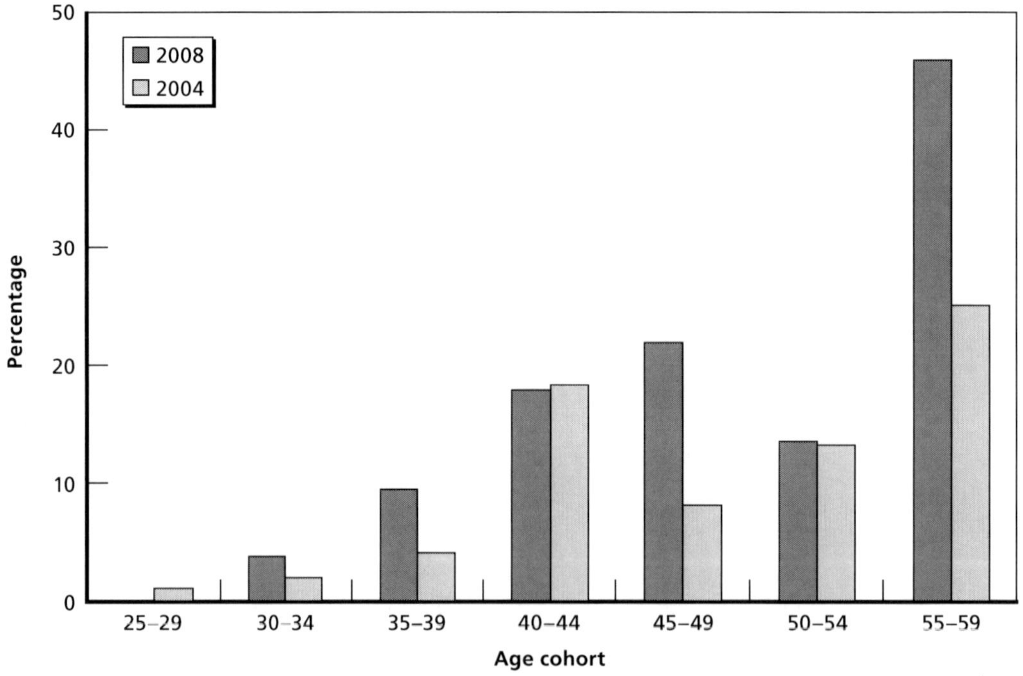

SOURCE: 2004 data are from Ministry of Planning and Development Cooperation, 2005.

RAND *TR715-2.12*

CHAPTER THREE

Employment

Survey Results

Figure 3.1 shows the percentage of individuals within each age cohort who are working. In June 2008, heads of household in al-Anbar appeared to enjoy what would be, by U.S. definitions, full employment. No female claimed to be working before age 23, and no male claimed to not be working by age 24. In other words, unemployment was confined to young males.[1]

Figure 3.2 contains similar information for December 2006, as reported retrospectively by individuals participating in the 2008 survey. The charts presented in Figures 3.1 and 3.2 look similar. In Figure 3.1, the May 2008 graph, every male age 24 and older has a job. In the

Figure 3.1
Percentage of Individuals with Jobs, by Age (May 2008)

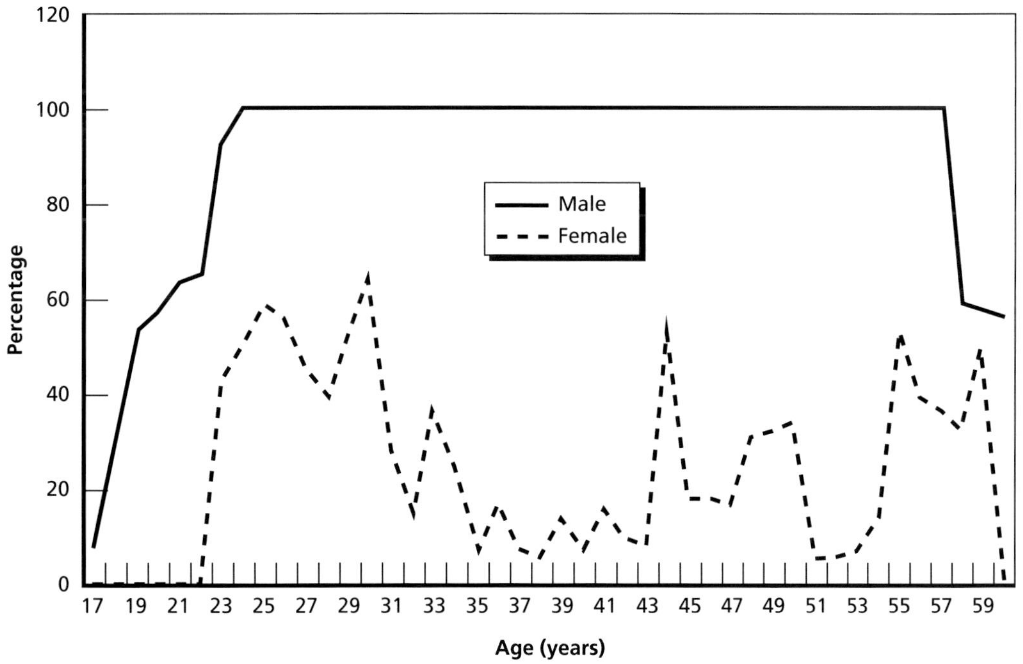

RAND *TR715-3.1*

[1] This and many other survey questions received 100 percent responses, where figures in the high 90s may have been more credible. Improvements were made in the follow-on questionnaire for 2009 submission to increase the fidelity of the answers from a statistical perspective.

Figure 3.2
Percentage of Individuals with Jobs, by Age (December 2006)

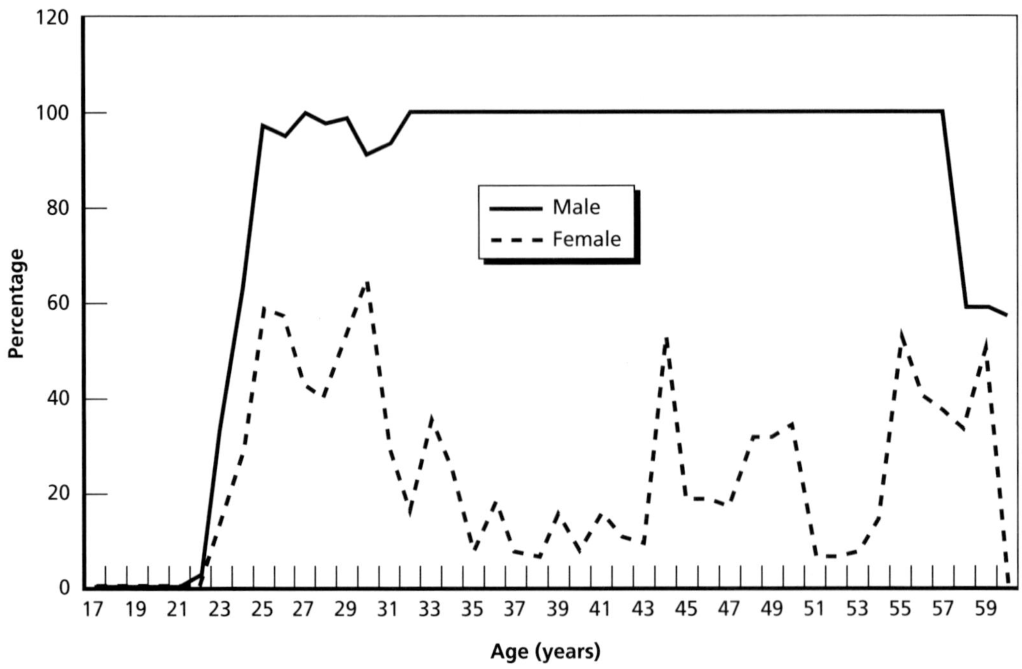

RAND *TR715-3.2*

December 2006 graph, almost every male age 25 and older (98.8 percent, or all but 17 of them) has a job. (Bear in mind that the 25-year-olds of the 2008 survey were 17 months younger in December 2006.) Incidentally, everyone who had a job in December 2006 had one in May 2008.

The big difference was the employment status of males ages 17–23 at the time of the 2008 survey. Of the 886 in that group, only 37 had jobs in December 2006; however, 438 had jobs in May 2008, a huge difference even when taking into account the 17-month difference in age. U.S. assistance may be partly responsible for this tight labor market. A number of Anbaris (18,000–20,000) associated with the Awakening movement have been hired as police. Hiring young male Iraqis as police has not only provided those individuals with employment, it has also meant that the remaining young men face less competition for work in the private sector. In addition, U.S. funding from the Commander's Emergency Response Program (better known as CERP) and other sources has paid for the construction of infrastructure and public buildings in al-Anbar, thereby increasing demand for labor. Not all of the increases in work can be traced to U.S. programs, however. The improvement in the province's security situation, which has resulted in a surge in private-sector activity, may be a more plausible explanation for increased employment, especially because the percentage of individuals working for the government is not particularly high.

Urban-rural distinctions among employment rates are modest. Males ages 20–24 have a 78-percent employment rate in both urban and rural areas. The employment rate among those ages 15–19 is 20 percent in towns and 17 percent in rural areas.

By way of comparison, Figure 3.3 contrasts the labor-force participation rate in 2008 with statistics from 2004.

Figure 3.3
Labor-Force Participation Rates, 2008 Compared with 2004

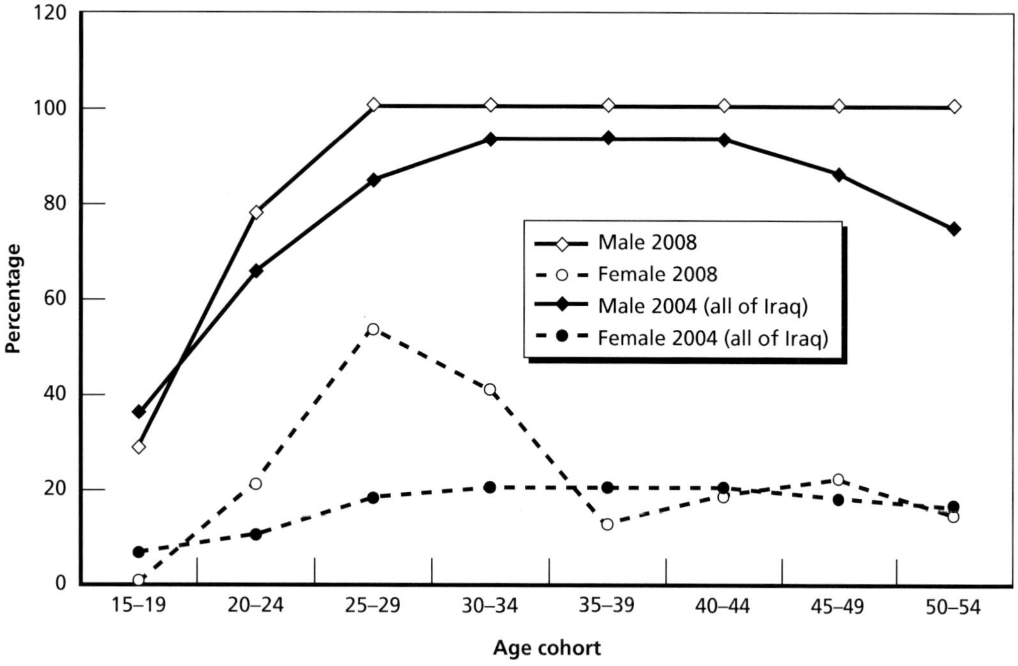

SOURCE: 2004 data are from Ministry of Planning and Development Cooperation, 2005.
RAND *TR715-3.3*

Because the 2008 survey shows that these young people eventually find work, the Iraqi government and U.S. assistance programs should be focused on training rather than employment generation. This focus will help raise the potential lifetime earnings of these young people by providing them with better skills.

Figure 3.4 shows the number of income earners reported per household. Every household has at least one income earner. Almost half have more than one. A few have as many as eight, although this is not visible in the figure.

Among the roughly 8,000 individuals who live in the 1,200 households surveyed, 217 can be categorized as both wanting to work and unemployed. Dividing this number by the total number who work or who stated that they wished to work yields an unemployment rate of 8.3 percent, the same recorded for al-Anbar by the 2004 survey *before* the extreme levels of violence experienced in 2005 and 2006. Every unemployed person in the 2008 survey is male; of these, 120 live in urban areas and 97 live in rural areas. In 18 of the households with an unemployed member, two people reported that they are seeking jobs. In 181 of the households with unemployed members, only one person reported looking for a job. Figure 3.5 gives the age breakdown of the unemployed.

Of the 217 people who are unemployed, 107 have asked friends and relatives for jobs, 54 have sought work with potential employers, 44 have registered at the local labor office, 57 have tried to start their own business, 59 have looked for work with nongovernmental organizations (NGO)s, and one admitted to doing nothing. Another 37 checked no boxes, not even the "did nothing" box.

Figure 3.6 displays the distribution of young men among the following three categories: those working, those who would like to work, and the rest.

Figure 3.4
Number of Households, by Number of Income Earners

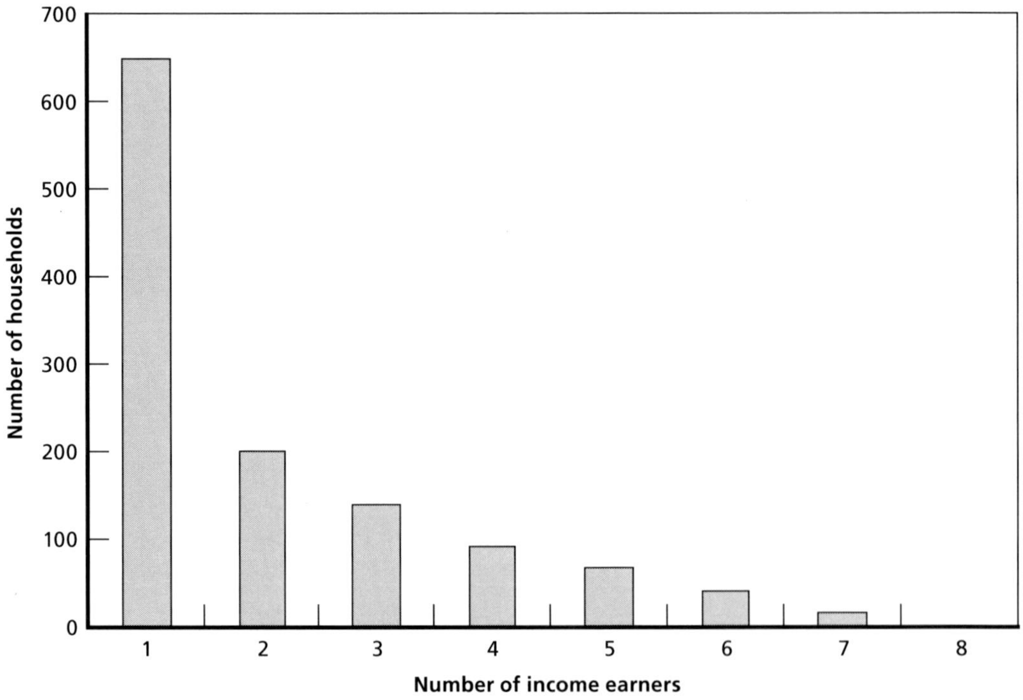

RAND *TR715-3.4*

Figure 3.5
Number of Unemployed Individuals, Ages 16–23, by Age

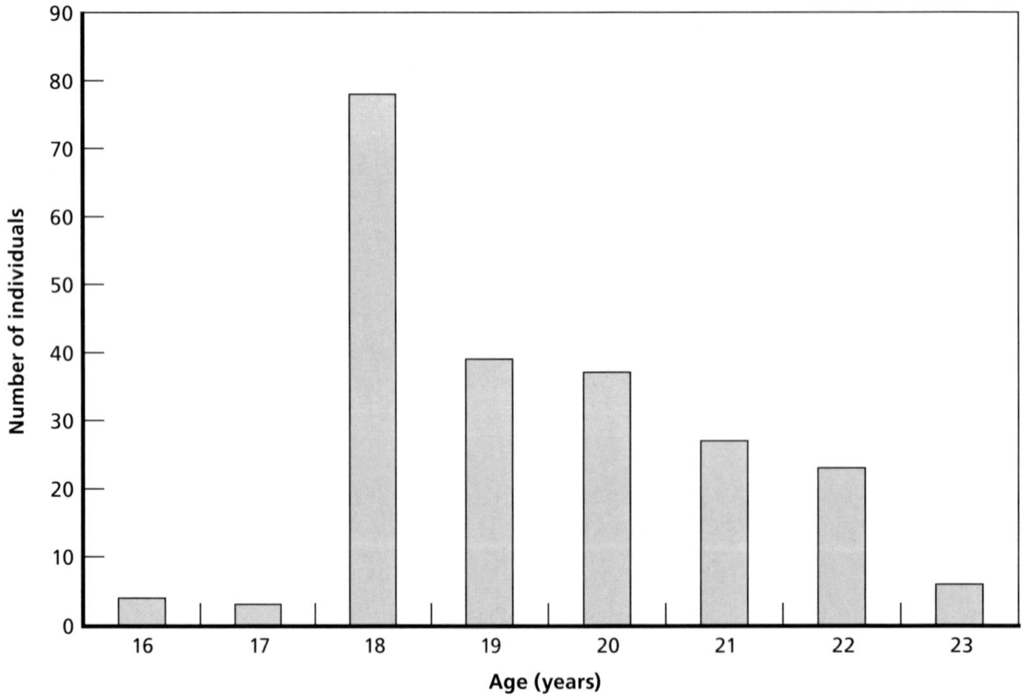

RAND *TR715-3.5*

Figure 3.6
Employment Status of Males, Ages 16–23, by Age

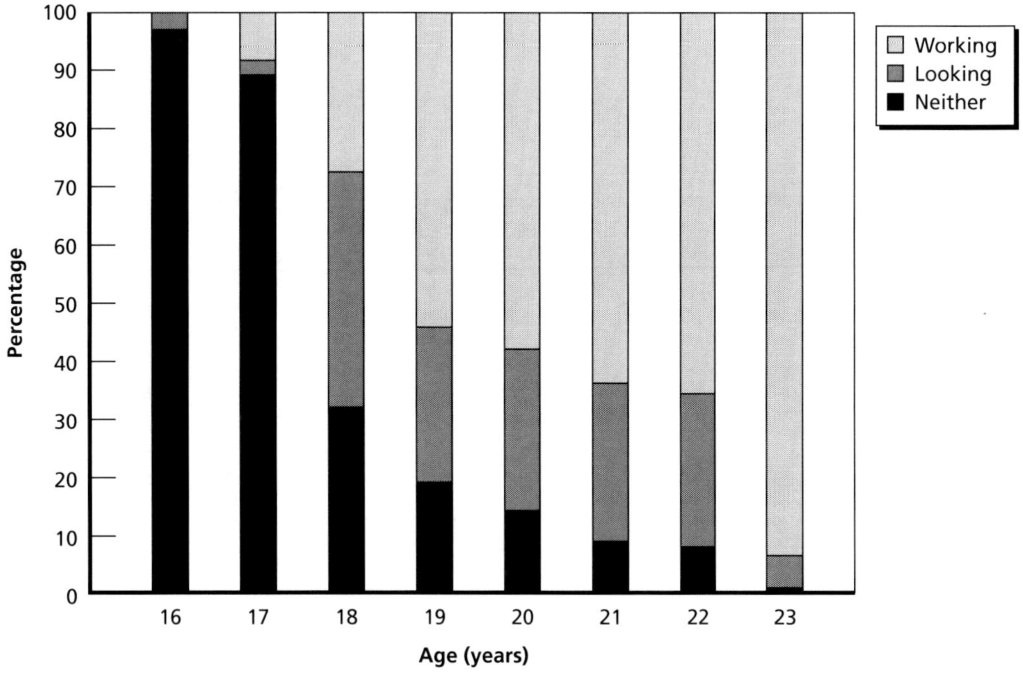

RAND *TR715-3.6*

Overall, the labor-force participation rate among males age 15 and older is 75 percent; the 2004 survey's figure was 66 percent. Similar changes are found for females: 23 percent in 2008 versus 17 percent in 2004. Both the male and the female participation rates reveal a substantially higher percentage of people in the workforce in 2008 compared with 2004. Because labor-force participation ratios tend to rise when times are good, these figures suggest that the economy has substantially improved. In general, al-Anbar's 2008 labor-force participation rates are on par with those of neighboring countries, except Turkey and Syria, where they are higher.

These results are in sharp contrast to much media reporting on Iraq, which cites very high rates of unemployment. However, all surveys in Iraq, like the 2004 survey and others that use large, randomly selected samples, have found results similar to those of the 2008 survey. In all of these surveys, as in ours, actual unemployment rates are a third or less of the figures cited by government officials and reported in the media, which often range from 40 percent to 50 percent. In a society where there is no safety net apart from the Public Distribution System, which provides food rations, necessity forces people to make money one way or another. In most instances, people opt for casual work or self employment. The discrepancy between claims by Iraqi government officials and the results of all large-scale surveys that used random sampling and standard international definitions of *unemployment* may be due to differences in definitions: Iraqi government officials may equate employment with a salaried (i.e., government) job and ignore most private-sector employment.

As many as 388 respondents answered "yes" to the question, "During the past week, did you want to work more hours?" Figure 3.7 lists the reasons why the respondents did not work more hours. Note that respondents were permitted to select more than one reason.

Figure 3.7
Why Respondents Who Wish to Work More Hours Have Been Unable to Do So

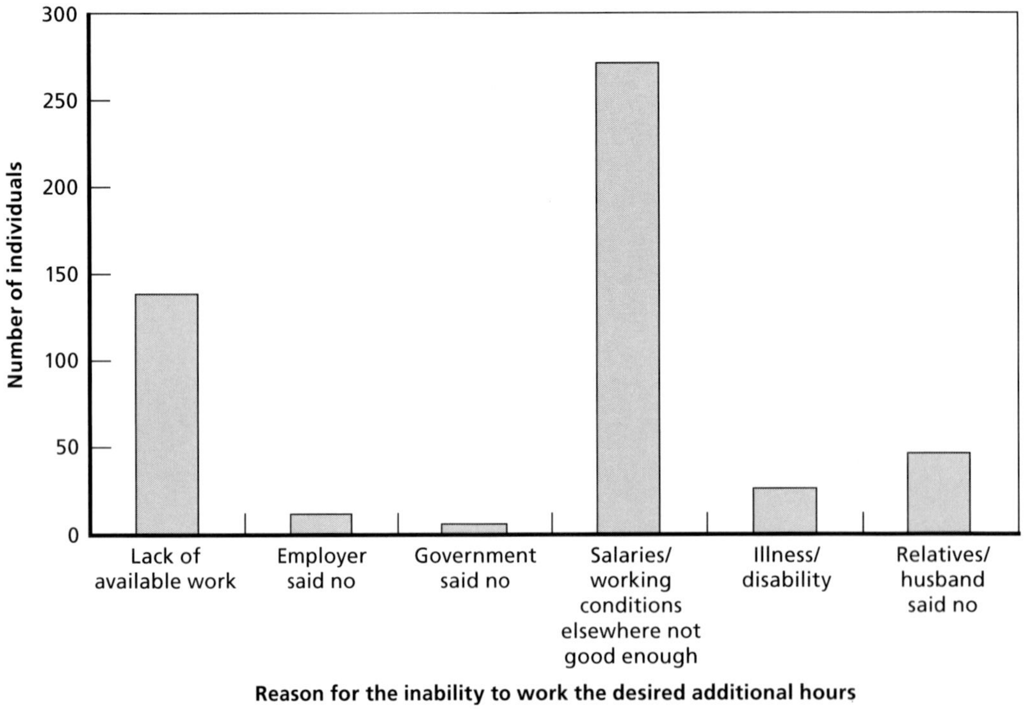

RAND *TR715-3.7*

However, self-reporting is a poor way of estimating underemployment. Respondents who stated that they wished to work more hours already worked more hours—44, on average—than those who said they had no desire to work more hours. Twenty percent of employed household heads said they would like to work more; by contrast, only 10 percent of other employed individuals said so. The places of work of those who said they would like to work more hours were smaller on average (employing an average of 7.9 people) than those of respondents who did not wish to work more hours (employing an average of 9.3 people). Finally, only 177 of the 388 (46 percent) who wanted more work actually actively sought more work.

One way to assess the nature of employment is to ask respondents whether they are employees of nonfamily businesses, employees of family businesses, employers of non–family members, or self-employed (a category that includes employers of family members). Table 3.1 shows the results of this question when asked during the 2008 survey.

It appears from the responses that Anbaris and Americans interpret some employment concepts in different ways. For example, among respondents who identified themselves as self-employed or employers of family members only, the average number employed in the enterprise was over six. Perhaps the number is so high because such individuals employed many family members; on the other hand, no respondents identified themselves as being employed by family members, leading to the possibility that many people who identify themselves as self-employed are really employed by family members. So, this observation remains interesting, as does the fact that all 412 people who identified themselves as self-employed are male. Otherwise, the key distinction is between those who work for establishments (i.e., those who are "paid employees") and everyone else. The former are more likely to be urban, are on average more than 10 years younger than the entire cohort of workers, work 10 percent fewer hours, and earn 30 percent less.

Table 3.1
Characteristics of the Self-Employed, Employers, and Employees

	Employment Category		
Characteristic	**Self-Employed[a]**	**Employer**	**Paid Employee**
Total	412	1,008	1,095
Urban	219	509	628
Rural	193	499	467
Male	412	724	891
Female	0	284	204
Age (years)	38.8	38.9	25.7
Hours worked (average)	45.3	45.3	41
Weekly salary (dinars)	104,915	116,835	79,311
Employees in the business (average)	6.2	2.9	20.3

[a] Includes those who employ family members exclusively and those employed by family members.

Another way of cutting the data is to ask individuals what kind of institution they work for: private, various forms of government, NGO, or other (e.g., the U.S. military). The results, shown in Table 3.2, reveal that the vast majority of workers work in the private sector. Again, the urban-rural distinction is not significant. Female participation in the state sector (i.e., state-owned firms and the local government) and in NGOs is significantly higher than in private firms. The Iraqi Army employs no women surveyed. Consistent with the tendency for older workers to employ themselves, the average age of those working for private firms is significantly higher than in any other employment category. Employees of state-owned firms and local governments work fewer hours than employees in other categories. Employees of the Iraqi Army work a standard 54-hour week. Wages are lower for employees of state-owned firms compared with other categories and higher for those in the Iraqi Army.

Figure 3.8 shows another way to slice the employment pie. It shows responses to the question, "What kind of work is this individual doing on the job?" Interestingly, individuals who identify themselves as farmers are age 57, on average. Individuals who identified themselves as tailors (70 percent of whom are female) are age 38, on average. People who identify themselves as workers are age 23, on average.

The long road corridors in al-Anbar, which run to Jordan and Syria, help keep the province's transportation sector relatively healthy, but al-Anbar tends to hold the short stick when it comes to government contracting and government employment. This is evident in the share of respondents who reported that they hold government jobs.

The rate of female employment in the private sector is much lower than that of male employment. The paucity of female workers has more to do with low labor-force participation rates than with the lack of jobs. Cultural norms hold that females should not work in the private sector. Families fear that women will be exploited and harassed, given the general instability, the failure to enforce labor regulations, and the general breakdown in the rule of law. Tribal traditions and religious beliefs further restrict job opportunities for females. Moreover, most females living in rural areas are unofficially employed in their families' businesses, including

Table 3.2
Characteristics of the Employed, by Type of Employer

	Employer Category					
Characteristic	Private Sector	State-Owned Firms	Local Government	NGOs	Other	Iraqi Army
Total	1,919	393	90	66	40	7
Urban	1,011	231	53	34	22	5
Rural	908	162	37	32	18	2
Male	1,635	259	52	34	40	7
Female	284	134	38	32	0	0
Age (years)	34.5	29.1	27.0	27.4	29.0	30.6
Hours worked (average)	45.2	35.9	35.6	44.2	44.6	54.0
Weekly salary (dinars)[a]	101,000	85,000	87,000	105,000	112,000	150,000
Employees in the business (average)	4.6	19.9	23.8	37.7	26.8	62.9
Respondents looking for more hours	316	47	11	5	8	1

NOTE: Ministry of Planning and Development Cooperation, 2005, found that 62 percent of people who were employed worked in the private sector (vs. 76 percent in the 2008 survey); 29 percent in state-owned firms (vs. 16 percent in the 2008 survey); 0 percent in the local government (vs. 5 percent in the 2008 survey); 4 percent in NGOs (vs. 3 percent in the 2008 survey), and 5 percent in other, unspecified categories (vs. 2 percent in the 2008 survey). The 2005 survey found that the percentage of Anbaris working for the Iraqi Army was 0.

[a] Includes 18 respondents who worked in the private sector and 12 who worked for other employers who were paid in U.S. dollars.

Figure 3.8
Percentage of Job Type Held, by Occupation/Field

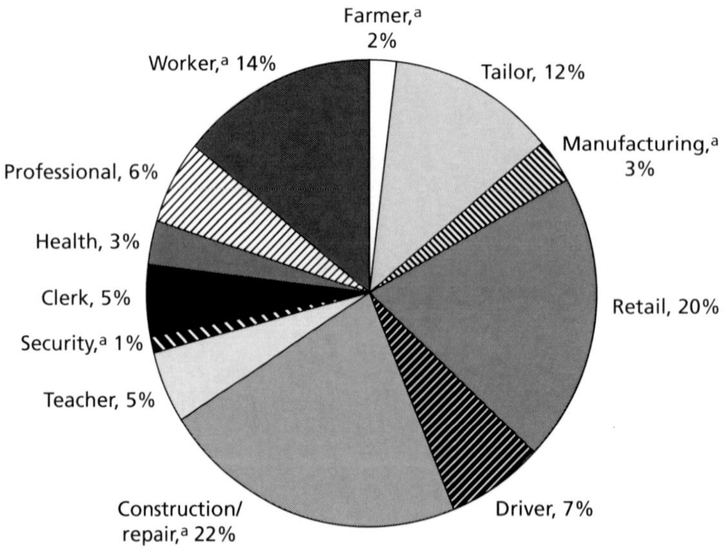

NOTE: The slices are arranged clockwise in descending order of the average age of the job holder.
[a] These occupations/fields happen to be manned exclusively by males.

RAND *TR715-3.8*

farming. The most-acceptable jobs for women outside family businesses are in the government and education. As in 2008, the 2004 survey found lower labor-force participation rates for females than for males; COSIT has found similar data in its own surveys. Female labor-force participation ratios have been dropping in Iraq, possibly due to the worsening economic conditions over the past three decades: Female labor-force participation rates dropped from 41 percent in 1977 to about 37 percent in 1997. In the 2008 survey, which measured mid-2008 rates, the rate was 26 percent.

CHAPTER FOUR

Income and Standards of Living

Background

Iraq's recent history of frequent wars has combined with large swings in oil revenues to create sharp fluctuations in average income and standards of living across the nation. Like many oil-exporting countries, Iraq experienced strong economic growth in the 1970s, attaining the status of a middle-income country due to increased oil exports and higher prices in the 1970s compared with the 1960s.[1] However, the Ba'athist regime's economic policies retarded economic growth by introducing severe economic distortions that fostered corruption while increasing economic inefficiency. Nevertheless, the regime did use part of the increase in oil income to expand access to public services.[2]

Iraq's economy was severely strained by the 1980–1988 Iran-Iraq War, the 1990–1991 Gulf War, and the subsequent sanctions regime. Although economic statistics were severely distorted during the 1990s, making it very difficult to measure even roughly changes in household incomes,[3] it is clear that standards of living deteriorated dramatically during this period, as did indicators of human development.[4] The share of the population living in poverty rose sharply.

Survey Results

Income

The data for this chapter are of two types. The first is earnings data for individuals, based on a pair of two-week intervals: one in May 2008 and one in December 2006. The second is data on household income (i.e., earnings plus transfers and sales of personal property). Households were surveyed to determine their income, by category, for two weeks in May 2008; their income, by category, for 2007; and their total income for 2006. The stories the data tell are mostly consistent from one period to the next, but they are not identical.

Each household was asked about the income earned by each employed individual during the most recent two-week period prior to the survey. The results show that incomes in al-Anbar

---

1 World Bank, "Iraq," Web page, copyright 2009.

2 Phebe Marr, *The Modern History of Iraq*, Boulder, Colo.: Westview Press, 2004, p. 164.

3 Amatzia Baram, "The Effect of Iraqi Sanctions: Statistical Pitfalls and Responsibility," *Middle East Journal*, Vol. 54, No. 2, Spring 2000.

4 World Bank, "Country Brief: Middle East & North Africa (MENA)—Iraq," August 2006.

rose sharply between 2007 and June 2008. Anbaris do not feel affluent, but half of them feel relatively comfortable, and there is a guarded optimism that conditions are likely to improve. The average overall income of employed individuals was just under 100,000 dinars (roughly $100, depending on exchange rates). Per-person rural weekly wages (averaging 99,100 dinars) and per-person urban weekly wages (averaging 98,100 dinars) were virtually identical. Of the 2,515 individuals who reported having earned some income, 30 were paid in U.S. dollars; the rest were paid in dinars. By contrast, no one reported having been paid in U.S. dollars 17 months earlier. This suggests the importance of U.S.-funded programs, some of which pay in U.S. dollars.[5]

Weekly incomes are clearly correlated with age (see Figure 4.1). On average, those under age 23 earn half of what their seniors make. Once they reach age 24, their incomes catch up with those of the rest of the adult community. Thereafter, there is slight correlation between age and earnings, but, on average, being a year older adds just under 1 percent to an individual's income. Data for December 2006 echo this relationship: Wages tended to rise slowly as a function of age. Note that the December 2006 line in the Figure 4.1 shows no statistics for those under age 23. This is because, as noted in Chapter Three, youths below that age rarely had jobs in 2006. Otherwise, the relatively weak correlation between age and weekly income is evident.

Figure 4.1
Weekly Income, by Age (May 2008 and December 2006)

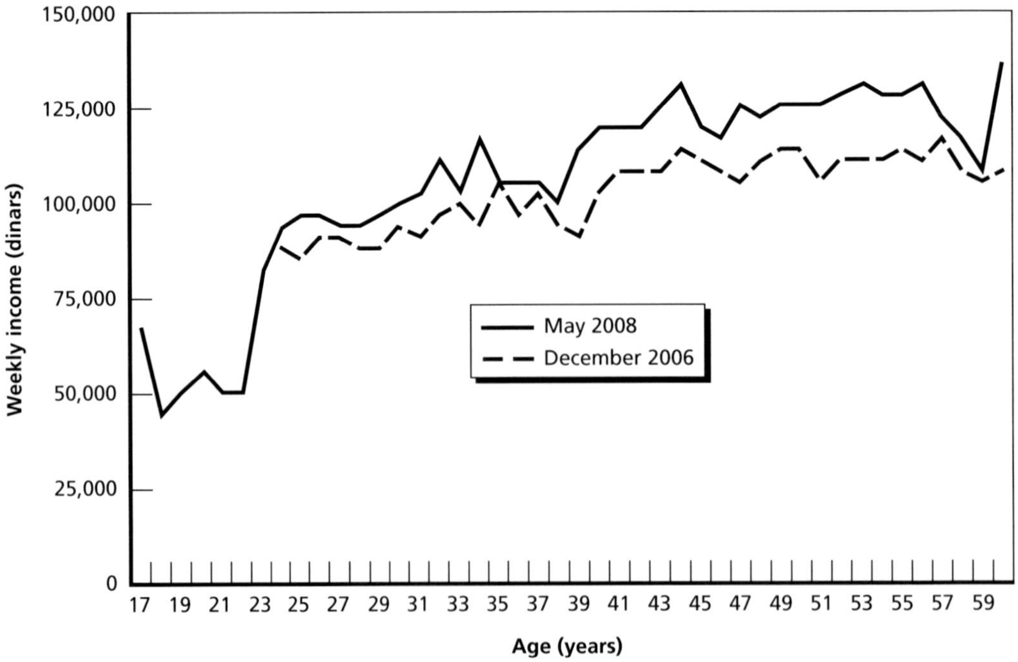

RAND *TR715-4.1*

[5] Among the 1,992 with jobs in December 2006, 289 could not remember what they had earned 17 months prior. Compared with those who remembered their income, people who forgot tended to be somewhat more rural, much less likely to be the head of a household (36 percent compared with 63 percent), more likely to be female, and younger (by four years).

In aggregate, weekly earnings went up 9 percent during the 17 months between December 2006 and May 2008. However, that aggregate conceals a wide variety of outcomes. Figure 4.2 illustrates the spread.

Wage rates for women are surprisingly close to those for men. Counting everyone, the average weekly wage is 97,400 dinars for men and 103,300 dinars for women.[6] When the large but low-wage and exclusively male cohort under age 23 is excluded, the wages for the remainder are 106,400 dinars for men and 103,300 dinars for women.

Urban-rural distinctions in *household* wages (i.e., the sum of wages of all household members) are not pronounced. On average, urban households have slightly higher aggregate wages (212,000 dinars) compared with rural households (200,000 dinars), but they also have more wage earners per household (2.17 vs. 2.02). The fact that household size in terms of its number of members was nearly identical (6.69 vs. 6.61) suggests that the modest difference in earnings may be due to better employment prospects in urban areas.

Anbaris derive income from a variety of activities, including work, transfers, renting property, and trading. In 2007, aggregated over all households, Anbaris received 55 percent of their income from earnings from labor, 6 percent from transfers, 9 percent from property rentals (including inheritances), and 30 percent from asset sales. During the two-week period in May 2008 studied during the survey, Anbaris received 65 percent of their income from earnings from labor, 8 percent from transfers, 17 percent from property rentals, and 10 percent from asset sales.

Figure 4.2
Distribution of Individual Earnings, by Increase/Decrease in Earnings Level Between December 2006 and May 2008

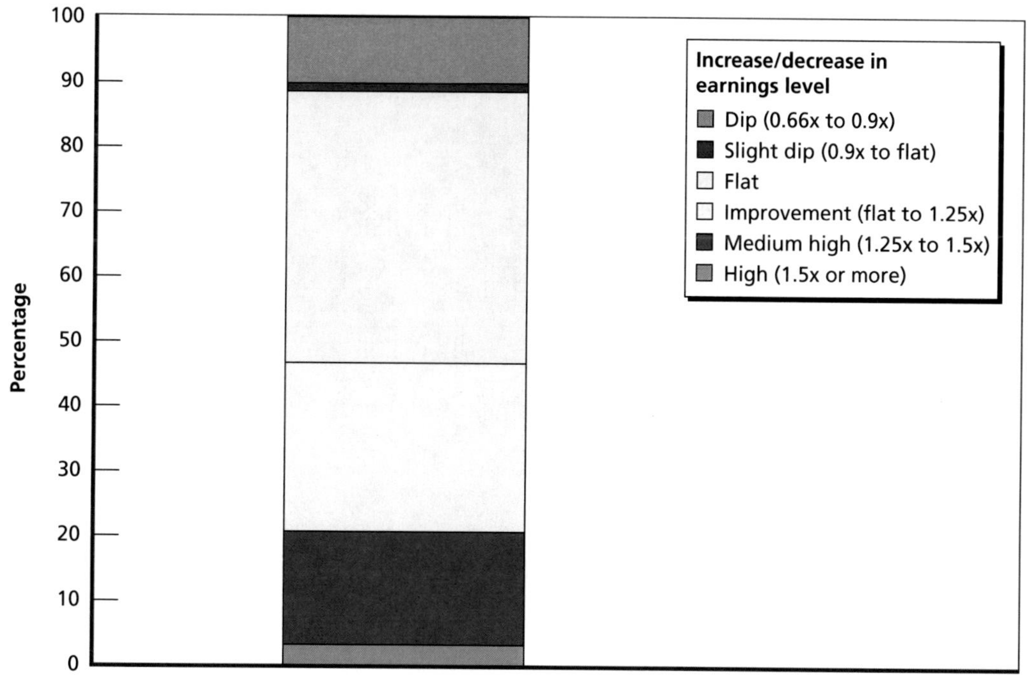

RAND *TR715-4.2*

6 As seen in Chapter Three, women are disproportionately employed by the government, state-owned enterprises, and NGOs—sectors where levels of salaried employment are much higher than in the private sector. These jobs also usually demand employees with skills that garner higher pay.

Insofar as some asset sales may be evidence of family distress, the decline in asset sales as a share of income may suggest that incomes in al-Anbar have risen across most households.

Figure 4.3 provides a breakdown of earnings by type of income. Wages account for a small portion of the pie. The largest sector is seasonal labor; taxi and other services (i.e., personal services) account for the second-largest slice.

Figure 4.4 shows similar share-of-earnings data for the whole of 2007. Income in-kind or from sales from gardens and other agricultural activities is important for most households.

Figure 4.5 provides another take on the data. It includes unearned income, such as transfers and property sales or rentals.

The heterogeneity of income sources is, of course, a characteristic of al-Anbar as a whole rather than of each Anbari household. For instance, Figure 4.6, which shows how many households receive income from particular activities, shows that no single source supplies more than 50 percent of the income of any of the 1,200 households.

In general, income-producing activities produced roughly 1 million dinars (about $1,000) in 2007 for each household that earned that type of money. Transfers per household were far smaller, but in 2007, at least, the small number of families (55) that did earn money by selling property realized an average of 20 million dinars (roughly $20,000).[7]

In 2007, most households got most of their money from earnings from labor, with almost 40 percent of all households receiving more than 90 percent of their income from this source (see Figure 4.7). This pattern held with even more force in May 2008.[8]

Figure 4.3
Share of Earnings, by Activity Type (May 2008)

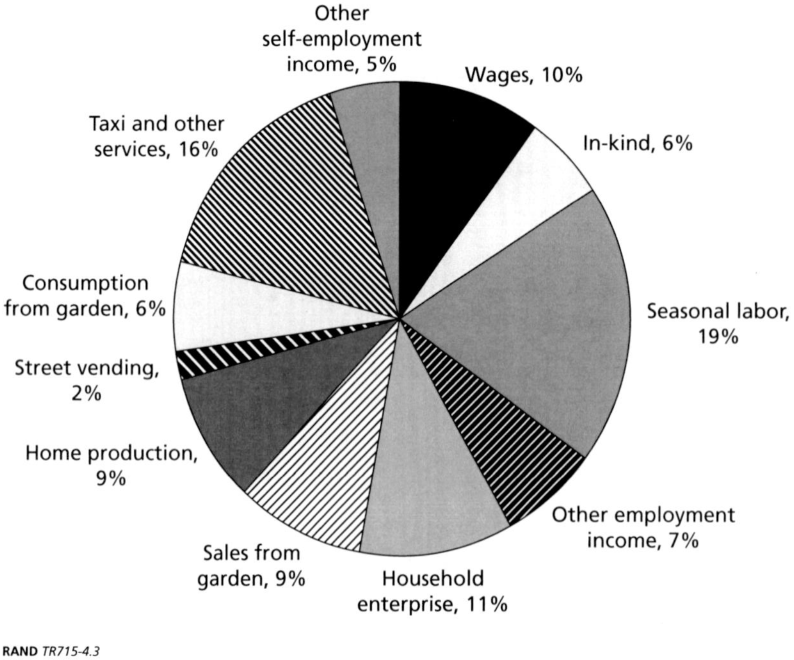

RAND *TR715-4.3*

[7] Iraqi families generally do not sell property to generate income unless they face straitened circumstances—e.g., a severe need for cash. Thus, high income from property sales may not be a sign of prosperity but rather the reverse.

[8] This may be an artifact of the infrequent nature of asset sales. In contrast to the 55 households who reported income from the sale of land or buildings, no household reported such income in the two-week period in May 2008.

Figure 4.4
Share of Earnings, by Activity Type (2007)

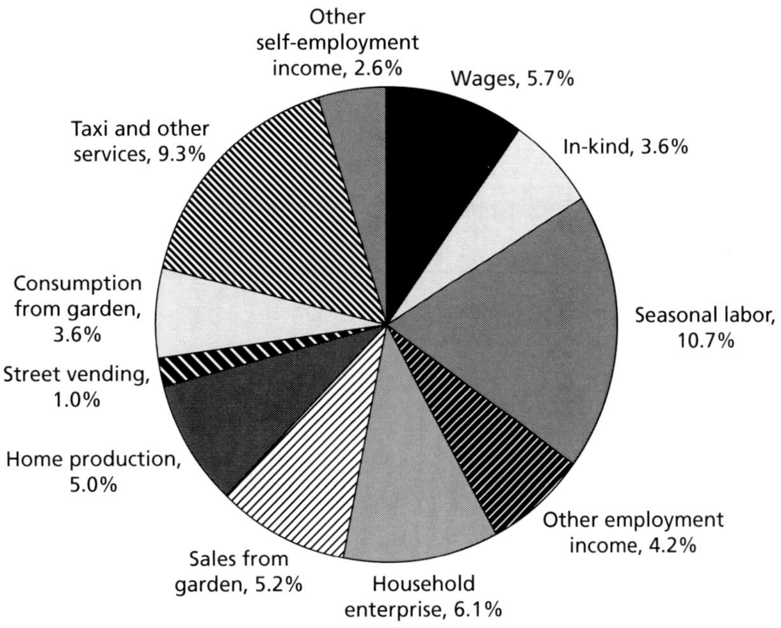

RAND *TR715-4.4*

Figure 4.5
Share of Income, by Activity Type (May 2008)

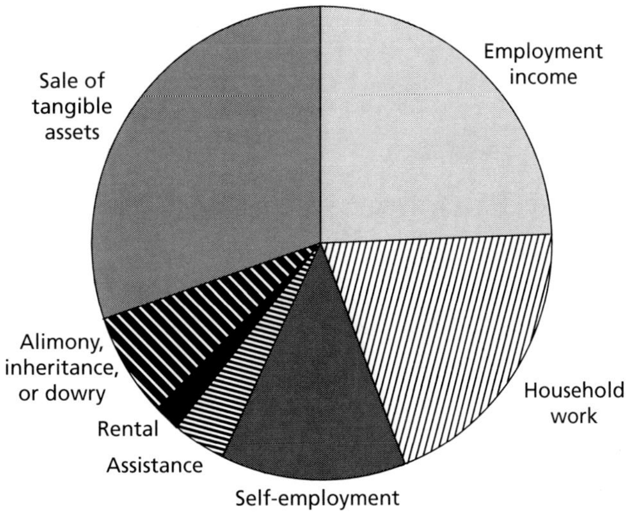

RAND *TR715-4.5*

Figure 4.6
Percentage of Households That Received Money, by Activity

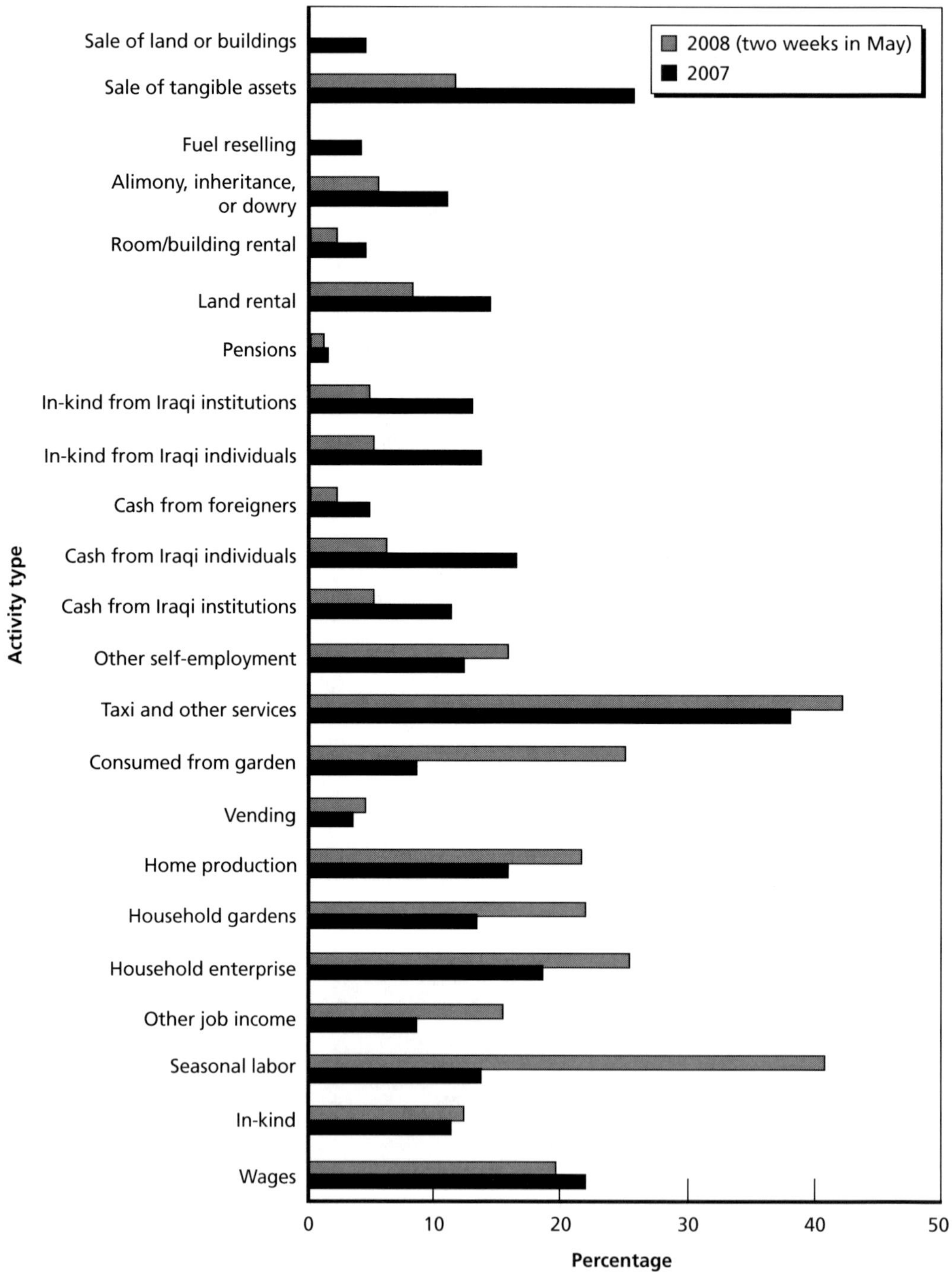

RAND *TR715-4.6*

Figure 4.7
Number of Households, by Labor Earnings as a Percentage of Total Income

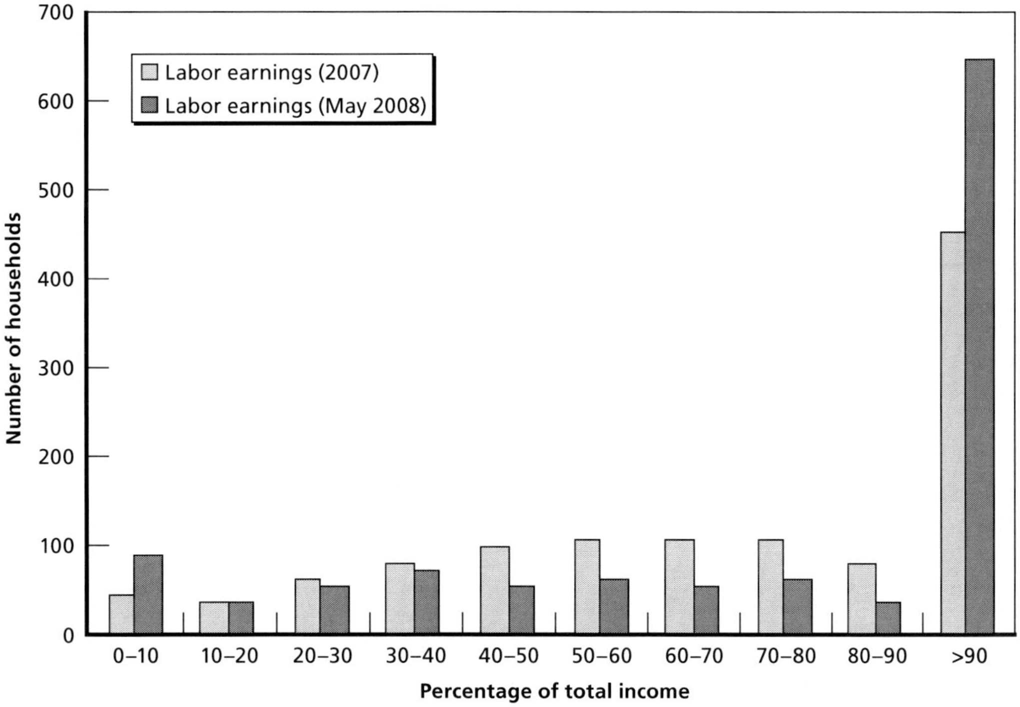

RAND *TR715-4.7*

Similar but opposite distributions characterize income from transfers (i.e., gifts), as shown in Figure 4.8. The large majority of Anbaris received less than 10 percent of their income from transfers in both the whole of 2007 and May 2008. Only 11 percent of all households received assistance: 5 percent from tribes, 4 percent from political groups, and 2 percent from other sources.

Transfers are the most likely means of ascertaining the potential role of insurgents and other violent actors in supporting Anbari households. Support from these groups (if accurately reported) would fall under "political groups" and "other sources." However, much of this assistance appears to come from political parties or legitimate NGOs in Anbar. These data suggest that, as of May–June 2008, considerably less than 6 percent of the population received income that might have come from violent groups

The definition of *transfers* (which were received by 40 percent of households) does not appear to include food rations, which were received by 92 percent of all households.[9] Every household that reported getting food rations received them from the Iraqi Ministry of Trade, picked them up at the local public-distribution site, and consumed them at home. Three-quarters of those receiving food rations acquired them within the last month; everyone else had received them within the last two months. For 90 percent of households, food rations are essentially money: Without them, they would have had to purchase the rations instead. Ten percent reported that they rely so heavily on food rations that they would have cut down on what they ate in the absence of rations.

---

[9] In Ministry of Planning and Development Cooperation, 2005, al-Anbar stands out as a province in which only 82 percent of all households received food rations. Compare this to the rate of 96 percent for the country as a whole.

Figure 4.8
Number of Households, by Transfers as a Percentage of Total Income

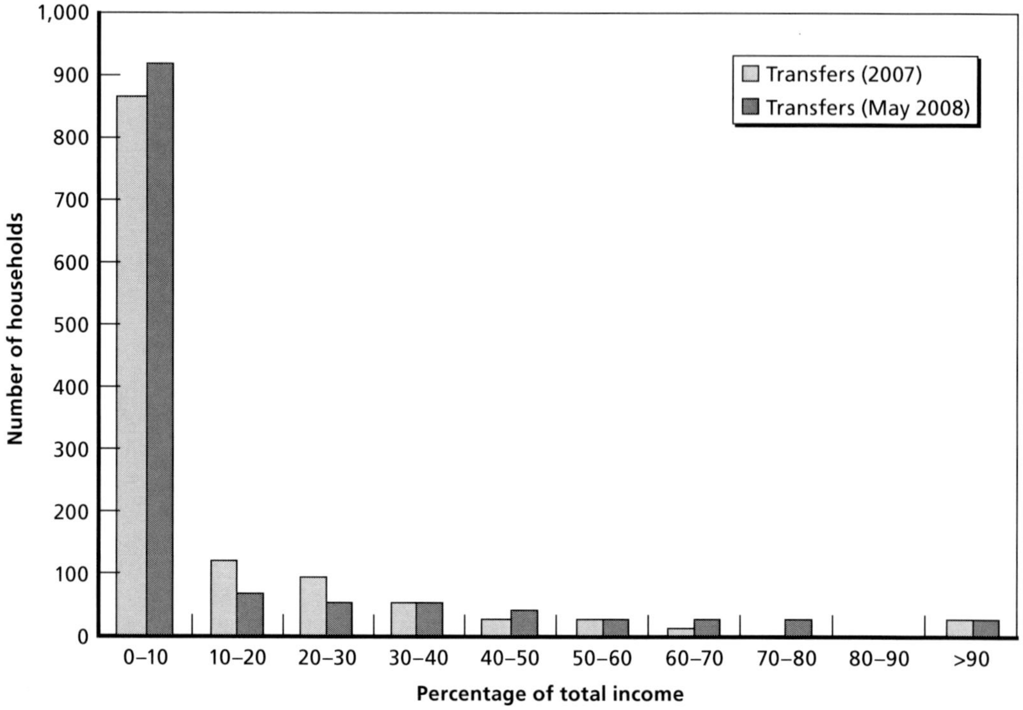

RAND *TR715-4.8*

In Figure 4.9, we examine the growth of income between 2006 and 2007; the growth in income per household is arrayed from the least growth to the most growth. Every household saw income growth of at least 17 percent, and most households saw substantial income growth (but some of the growth can be attributed to inflation).[10] The median increase was 50 percent.

Based on survey results, the distribution of income from all sources in al-Anbar seems to be fairly equal.[11] In 2006, the poorest half of Anbari households had incomes of 63 percent of the provincial average. In 2007, the poorest half had incomes of 73 percent of the provincial average.[12] Figure 4.10 illustrates the ratio between average provincial incomes and the incomes of the poorest 10 percent, the next-poorest 10 percent, and so on.

Finally, in Figures 4.11 and 4.12, we look at the influence of education on sources and levels of income. Contrary to expectations, higher education levels are not correlated with a high percentage of incomes arising from wages—or even higher incomes in general.

When measuring the percentage of income from a fixed monthly wages, as in Figure 4.12, the pattern is more distinct: Those with a college education receive almost 20 percent of their aggregate income from fixed monthly wages, while every other group except for the uneducated receive almost none of their income from fixed monthly wages.

---

[10] Inflation in 2006 and 2007 was high, hitting 50 percent year on year in some months (International Monetary Fund, *Iraq: Second Review Under the Stand-By Arrangement and Financing Assurances Review—Staff Report*, IMF Country Report No. 08/383, Washington, D.C., 2008, Table 1, p. 19).

[11] This may, however, be an artifact of sampling methods and income-group scaling.

[12] By way of contrast, data from the 1970 U.S. census show that similar figures for U.S. metropolitan areas in 1970 ranged from 41 percent to 53 percent.

Figure 4.9
Growth in Real Income Between 2006 and 2007, by Number of Households

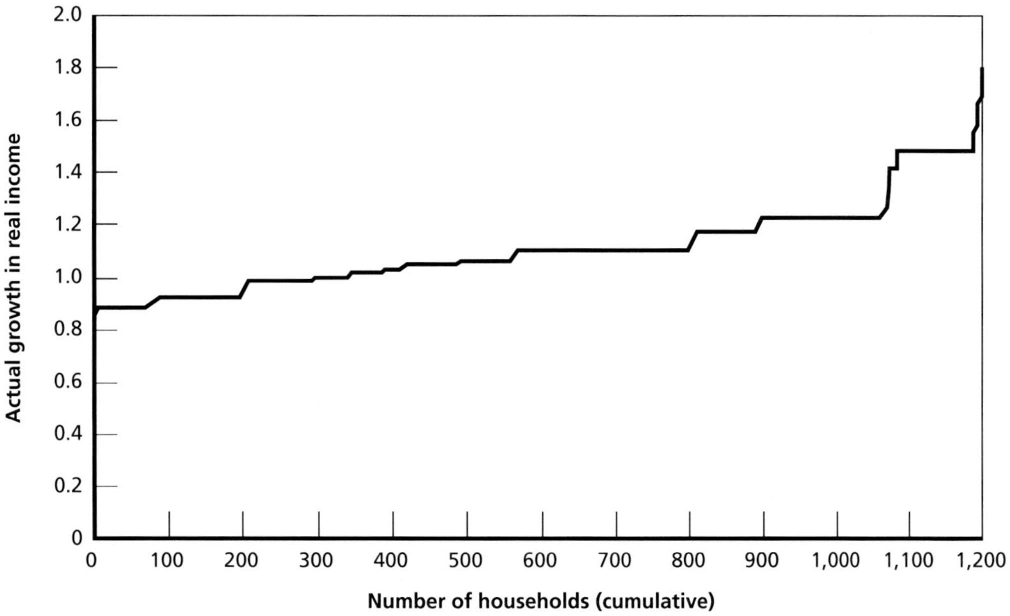

RAND *TR715-4.9*

Figure 4.10
Incomes as a Percentage of Average Incomes, by Decile (2006 and 2007)

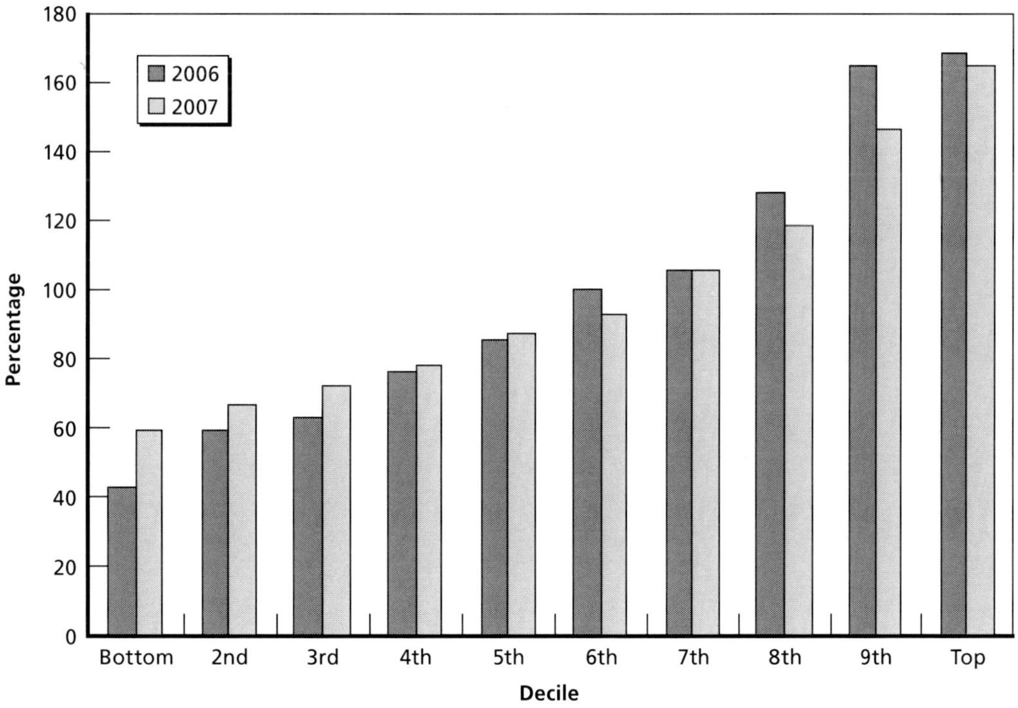

RAND *TR715-4.10*

Figure 4.11
Average Annual Income, by Type, by Education Level of Household Head

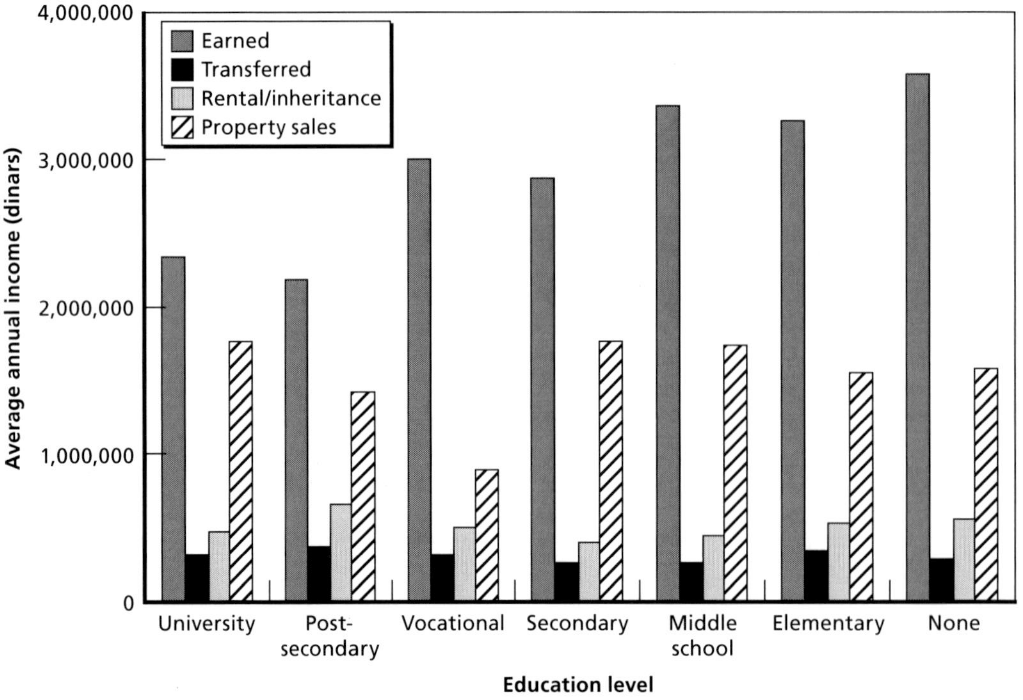

RAND *TR715-4.11*

Figure 4.12
Percentage of Income from Wages in 2007, by Education Level of Household Head

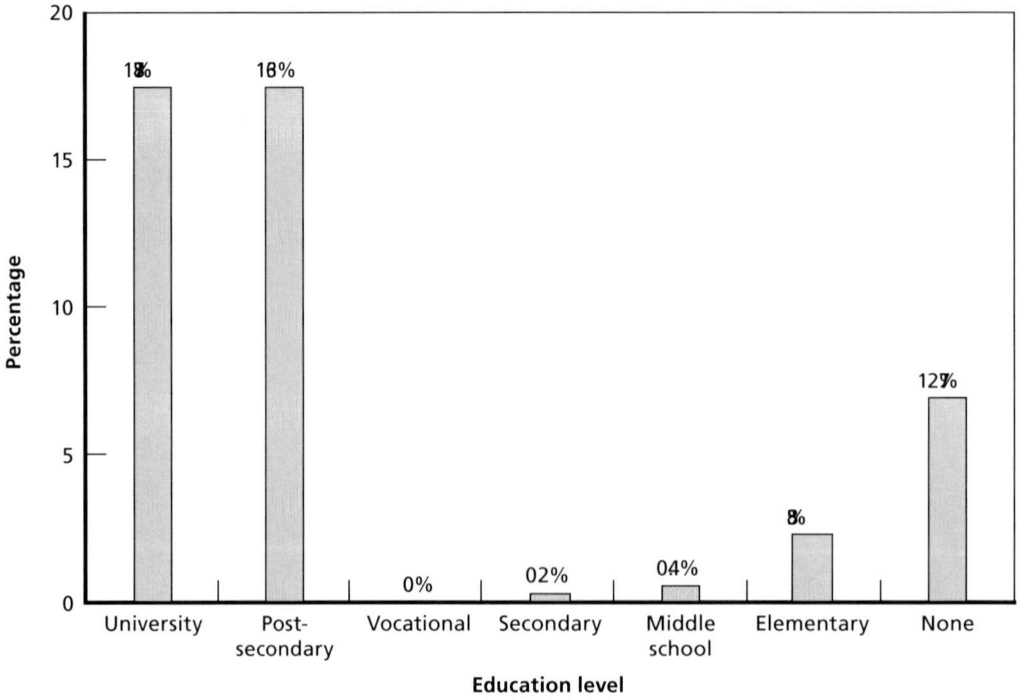

RAND *TR715-4.12*

Standards of Living

Table 4.1 shows how heads of household perceive their household's standard of living. As shown in Table 4.2, Anbaris are cautiously optimistic about the future of the economic situation

Two things seem most striking about these numbers: (1) the complete absence of household heads who identified their households as well-off and (2) the complete absence of household heads who are very confident that economic conditions will improve. The number of respondents who are fairly confident that the situation will improve is roughly equal to the number who were less or not at all confident. Whether all this represents actual conditions in al-Anbar or cultural pessimism cannot be determined. Half of the population thinks it lives well; the other half does not.

Based on questions about what households can afford, the typical Anbari household comes across as struggling but also possessing elements of Iraqi middle-class status. Most households say they can afford to eat a protein-rich meal every other day, pay for a funeral, provide adequate shelter for their family, purchase new clothes, and replace worn-out furniture and appliances (see Figure 4.13). Just under two-thirds believe they can start or expand their family (this, in a society whose birthrate is quite robust). Yet, more than half of the households surveyed experience problems affording fuel or power for adequate heating and cooling. Most households would have trouble buying some big-ticket items, such as weddings or vacations.

Anbaris, as a rule, do not have much in the way of savings. Just over 20 percent of all households have a bank account.[13] No household, according to the survey, uses a *jam'iyya,* a type of cooperative bank, to save money.

Table 4.1
Standard-of-Living Perceptions

Standard-of-Living Description	Household Heads Who Agree That the Description Fits Their Households (percentage)
We are well-off	0
We are not well-off, but we live well	49
We do not live well, but we are not poor	21
We are poor	30

Table 4.2
Confidence That the Economic Situation Will Improve

	Level of Confidence That the Economic Situation Will Improve (percentage)				
Reported Standard of Living	Very	Fairly	Not Very	Not at All	Don't Know
We are well-off	N/A	N/A	N/A	N/A	N/A
We are not well-off, but we live well	0	42	28	0	30
We do not live well, but we are not poor	0	36	30	12	22
We are poor	0	26	37	8	28

[13] The weakness of the banking sector arises, in part, from the 1990s, when the Iraqi currency depreciated sharply and those who had bank accounts lost the value of their savings. Iraqis view the purchase of big-ticket items, such as vehicles, real estate, or foreign currency, as a better way of saving money than using savings accounts. Foreign currency is usually kept in safe places in the home. Women may use jewelry, especially that made of gold, as a form of savings.

Figure 4.13
Percentage of Households That Can Afford a Particular Item

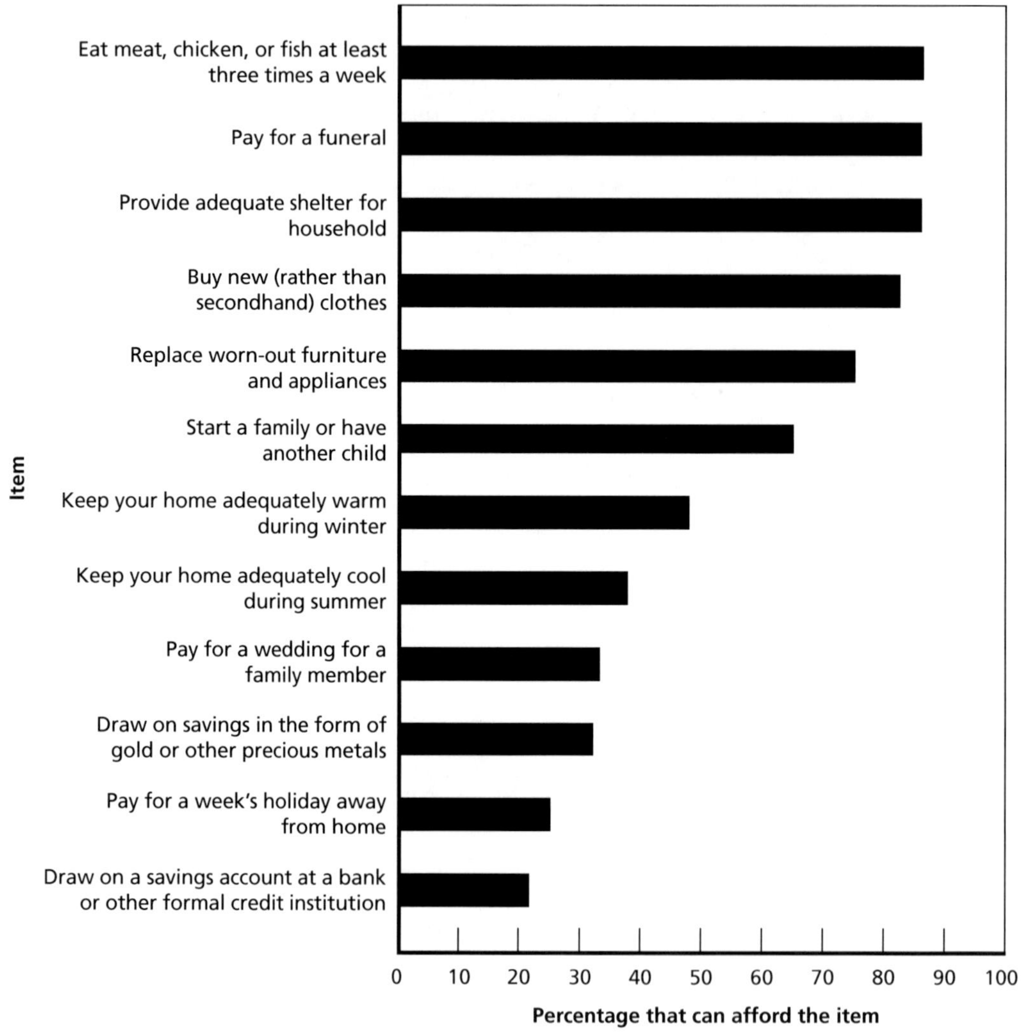

RAND *TR715-4.13*

This struggle to save money carries over into the ability to raise money quickly. When asked whether the household could get its hands on 200,000 dinars (roughly $200) within a week, roughly a third felt they had the resources to do so; a third felt they could, in effect, borrow the money; and a third felt they could not get the money (see Figure 4.14).[14] Over 30 percent of households have assets in the form of gold or other precious metals.

Although Anbaris are not affluent, the penetration of consumer durables into households is quite high (see Figure 4.15). Every household owns a stove and an oven, an electric fan, at least one radio/cassette player, a television set, and a satellite dish. Refrigerators and videocassette players are almost as ubiquitous. **Even personal computers and cars, quintessential symbols of affluence, can be found in half of all households.**

[14] In answer to a similar question asked by the Iraqi government in the 2004 survey about a somewhat smaller sum of money, 22 percent of Anbari households said they could raise the money, 46 percent would need help, and 32 percent had serious doubts they could do so.

Figure 4.14
Response of Households When Asked, "Could You Raise 200,000 Dinars in a Week?"

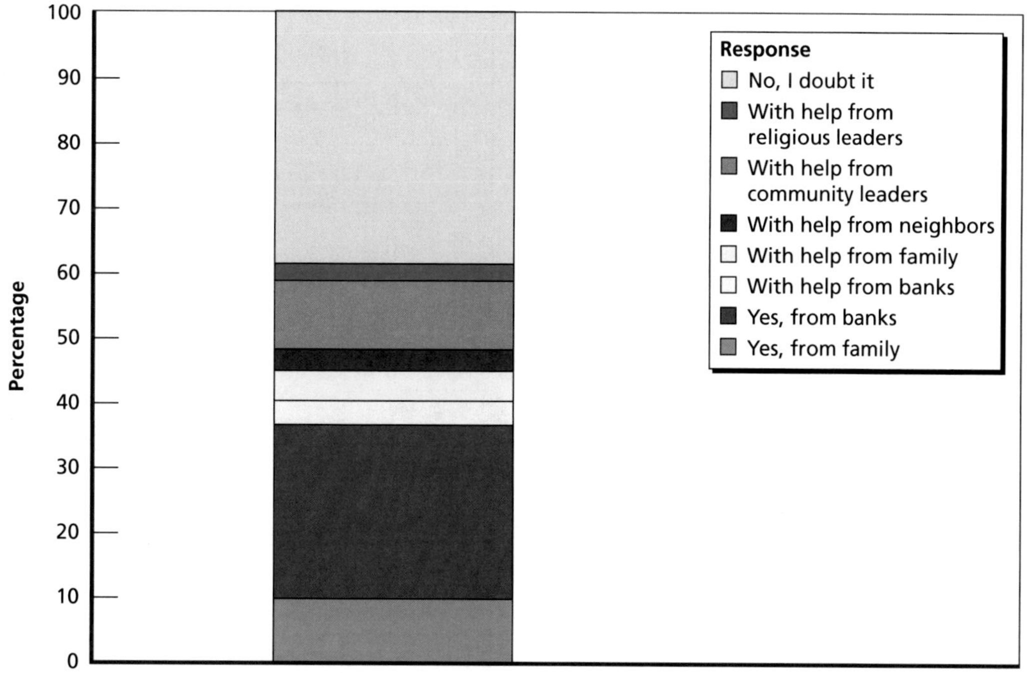

RAND *TR715-4.14*

Mobile phones have become increasingly characteristic of the developing world, where they are far more prevalent than landlines. Al-Anbar is no exception. Most Anbaris do not have landlines; most of those who do complained of unstable connections (see Figure 4.16). **By contrast, every household reports owning a cellular phone, and every household reports that its cellular-phone connections are stable.**

Although just over half of Anbari households have access to a personal computer, very few have their own Internet connections. Almost every household has some access to the Internet, but, for the most part, its members acquire access by visiting a cybercafé (see Figure 4.17). Indeed, owning a computer has only a modest effect on how people access the Internet.

Figure 4.15
Percentage of Households That Own at Least One of a Set of Household Items

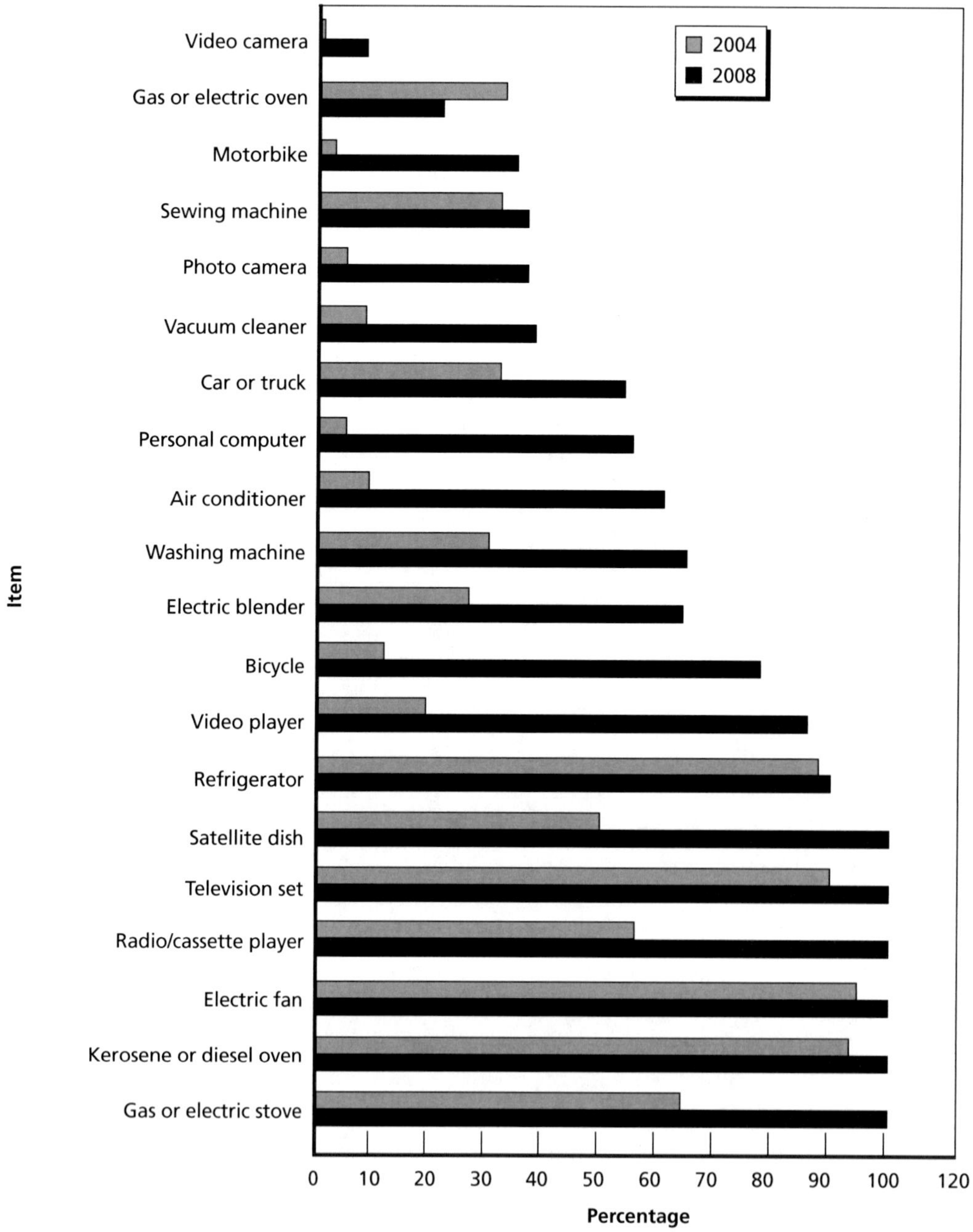

SOURCE: 2004 data are from Ministry of Planning and Development Cooperation, 2005.
NOTE: In 2008, some households indicated that they owned an item, but that it was broken; these items are counted as half an item each in this figure.
RAND *TR715-4.15*

Figure 4.16
Percentage of Households with a Landline Phone Connection

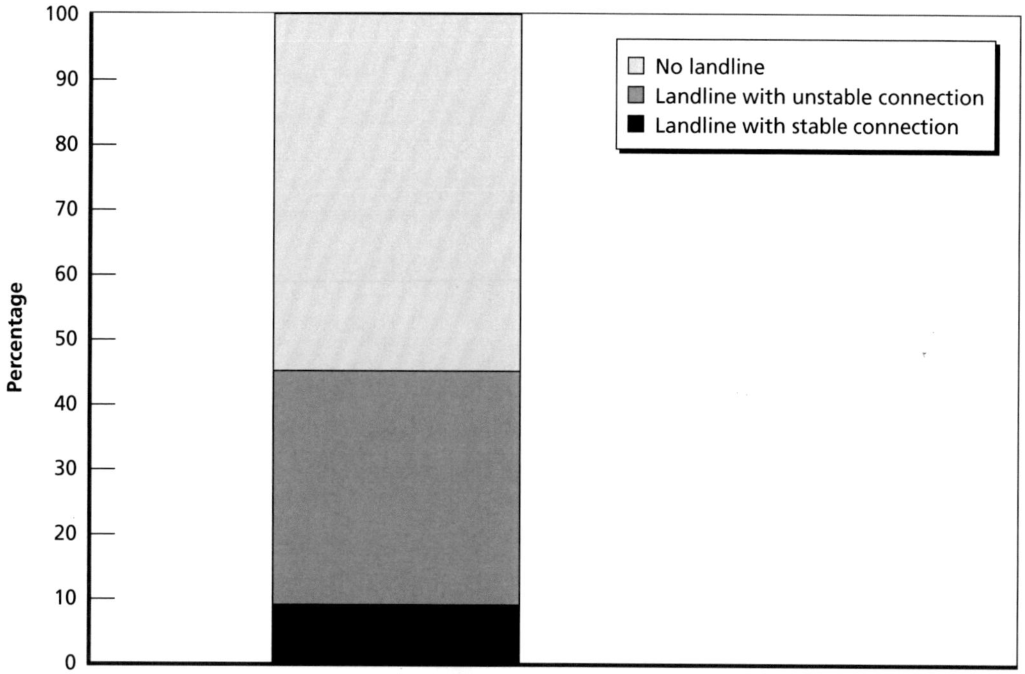

RAND *TR715-4.16*

Figure 4.17
How Households Access the Internet

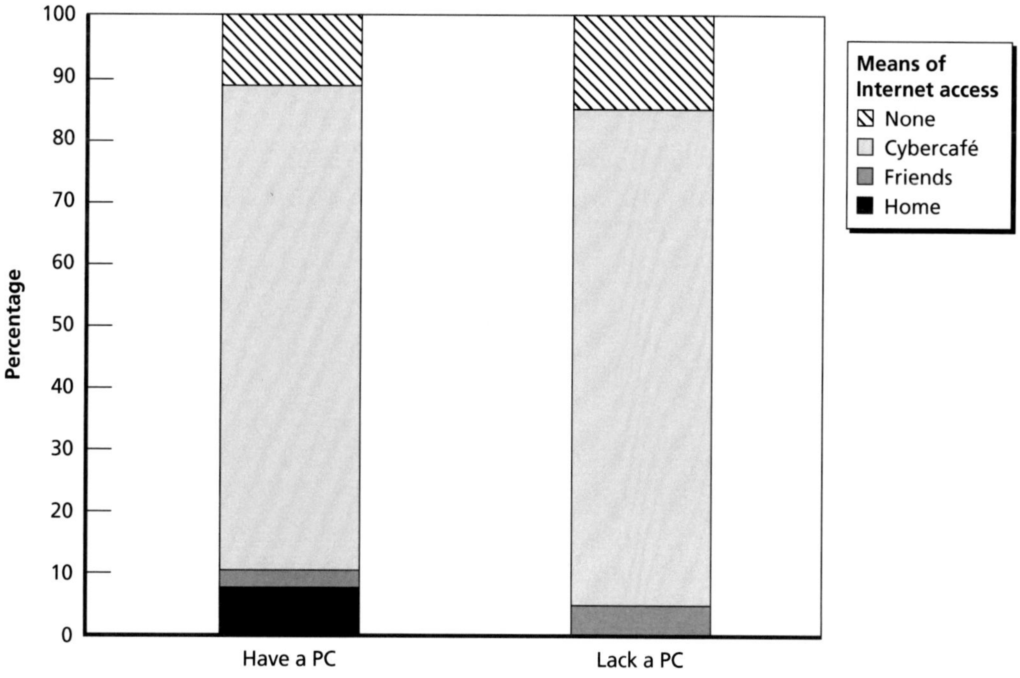

RAND *TR715-4.17*

CHAPTER FIVE

Education

Background

Iraq was once regarded as having one of the most developed educational systems among Arab countries. Before the Iran-Iraq War, the Iraqi government spent 6 percent of its gross domestic product and 20 percent of its total budget on education, spending an average of roughly $620 per student.[1] Tens of thousands of schools were built during the "golden age" of Iraq's educational system between the 1960s and the 1980s. According to the United Nations Educational, Scientific and Cultural Organization, before 1991, 100 hundred percent of Iraqis of elementary-school age were enrolled in school. The Iraqi system of higher education was internationally recognized. Following the first Gulf War, spending on education was cut sharply, resulting in the system's decline. After 1990, spending on education dropped to 8 percent of the total government budget; average spending per pupil fell to only $47 per year.[2]

Survey Results

According to the survey results, educational attainments are highly correlated with age (see Figure 5.1). Age 50 represents the breakpoint between widespread illiteracy and little or no education on the one hand and literacy and schooling on the other. Schooling of both sexes appears to be universal between the ages of 7 and 22.

Figure 5.2 provides a closer snapshot of the school-age population by type of school. In general, Iraqi children stay within their grade, graduating to the next level each year.

As Figure 5.3 indicates, many young men are enrolled in higher education. Of 752 youths ages 19–22, most of the males are in the labor force, but almost all of them attend school as well. Most females in this age group are also enrolled in higher education; however, women of this age rarely work.

When asked to supply the main reason why a particular household member has never attended school, some respondents cited the need to support their family economically or stay home and care for family members (12 percent). Six percent said they had no interest in school. Three percent were not enrolled in school due to their inability to access the school or to a lack of transportation. Three percent expressed concern about the safety of students, including girls (see Figure 5.4).

---

1 "Iraq, Education, and Children of Conflict," transcript of an April 8, 2008 conference at the Council on Foreign Relations, Federal News Service, Inc., 2008.

2 "Iraq, Education, and Children of Conflict," 2008.

Figure 5.1
Schooling, by Age

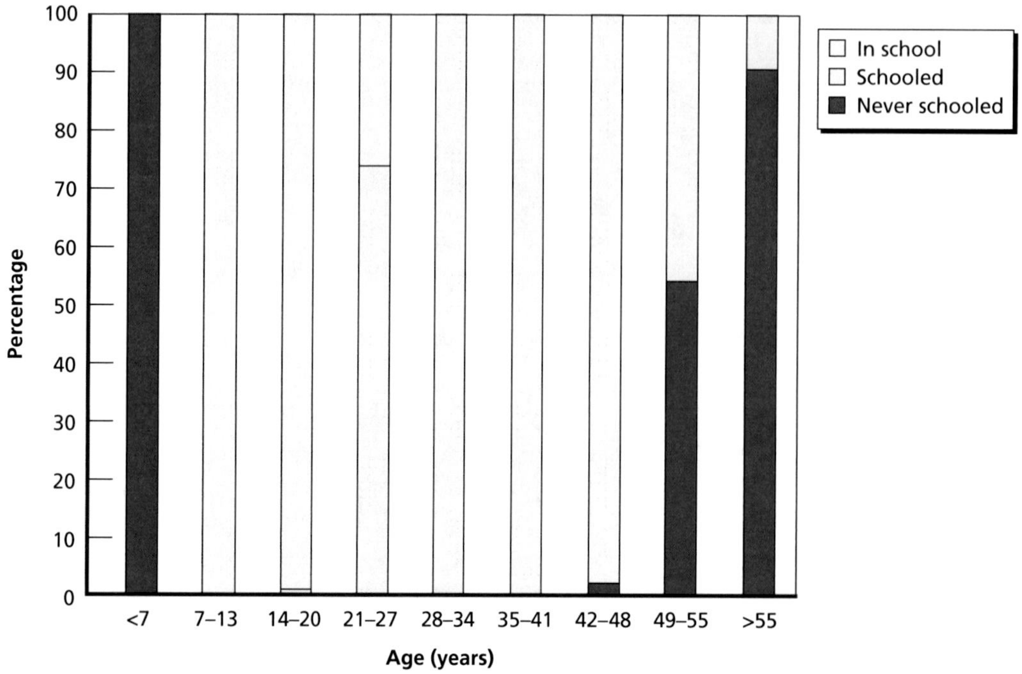

RAND *TR715-5.1*

Figure 5.2
School Attendance, by Type of School, by Age

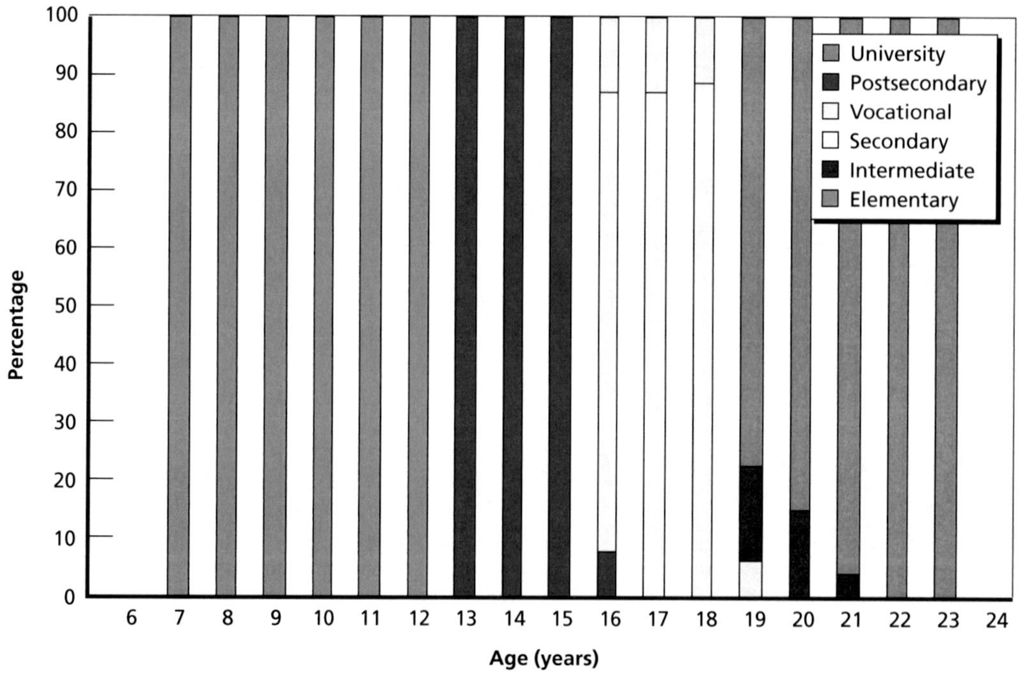

RAND *TR715-5.2*

Figure 5.3
Education and Employment Status of Males and Females, Ages 19–22

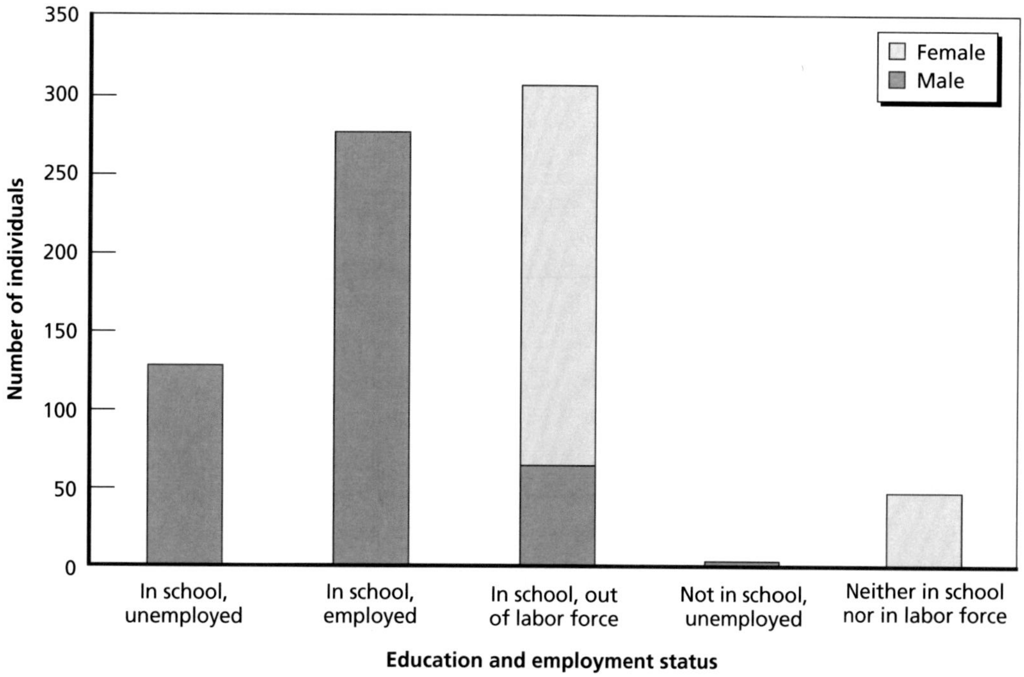

RAND *TR715-5.3*

Figure 5.4
Main Reason for Not Attending School, by Age

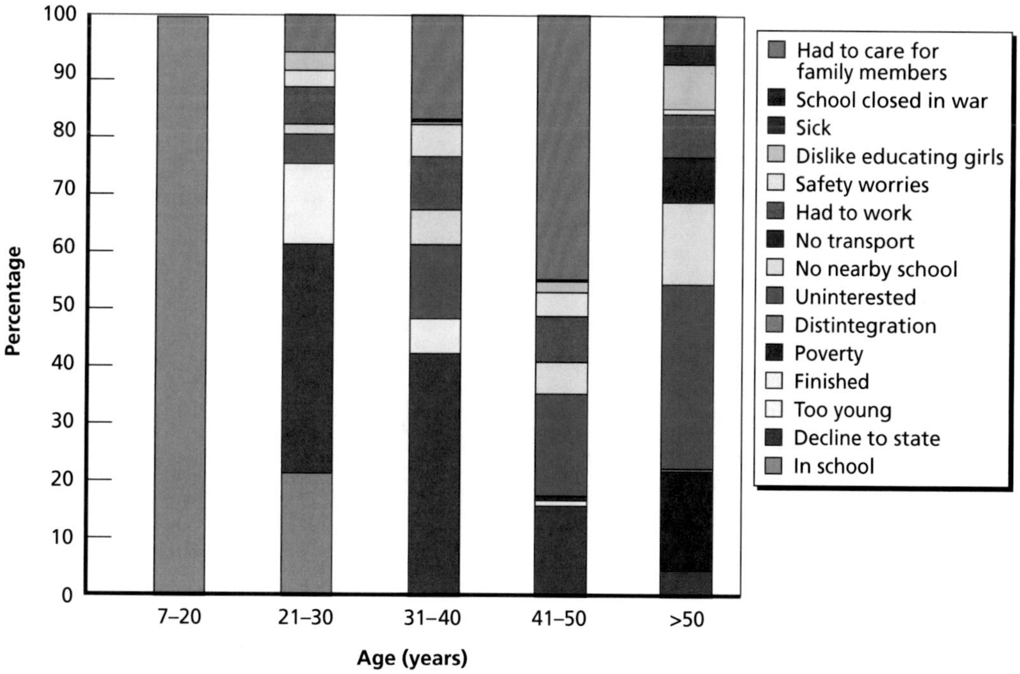

RAND *TR715-5.4*

Urban-rural distinctions do not seem to be correlated with educational attainment, as shown in Figure 5.5.

According to the survey, the Anbari population is literate. Large majorities (of 78 percent each) say they can either understand everyday written material or write a letter to friend. Survey respondents report that for Iraqis between the ages of 7 and 50, all males and all but 1.5 percent of females are able to read and write. For those over age 50, only a third of all males and a tenth of females were reported to be fully literate. This is an improvement over 2004 data, which showed that 75 percent of males age 15 and older and 52 percent of all females were fully literate. These figures contrast with some of the experiences of U.S. military personnel involved in training recruits for the Iraqi Security Forces. **A substantial share of applicants for jobs in the security forces fail basic literary tests. The difference is due to both self-reporting and differing definitions of *literacy*.**

As shown in Figure 5.6, household spending on education varies. About 13 percent of students cost less than 150,000 dinars (roughly $150) to educate. Nearly half (48 percent) cost 150,000–299,999 dinars (roughly $150–$300) to educate. Fewer than 10 percent cost more than 600,000 dinars (roughly $600) to educate. These amounts account for a substantial share of household expenditures. **Spending patterns indicated that education is given high priority in Anbari families.**

Not surprisingly, a household's expenditures on education vary depending on the age of the household's dependents (see Figure 5.7). They rise in step-like fashion with the transition

Figure 5.5
Education Level of Household Heads, by Region

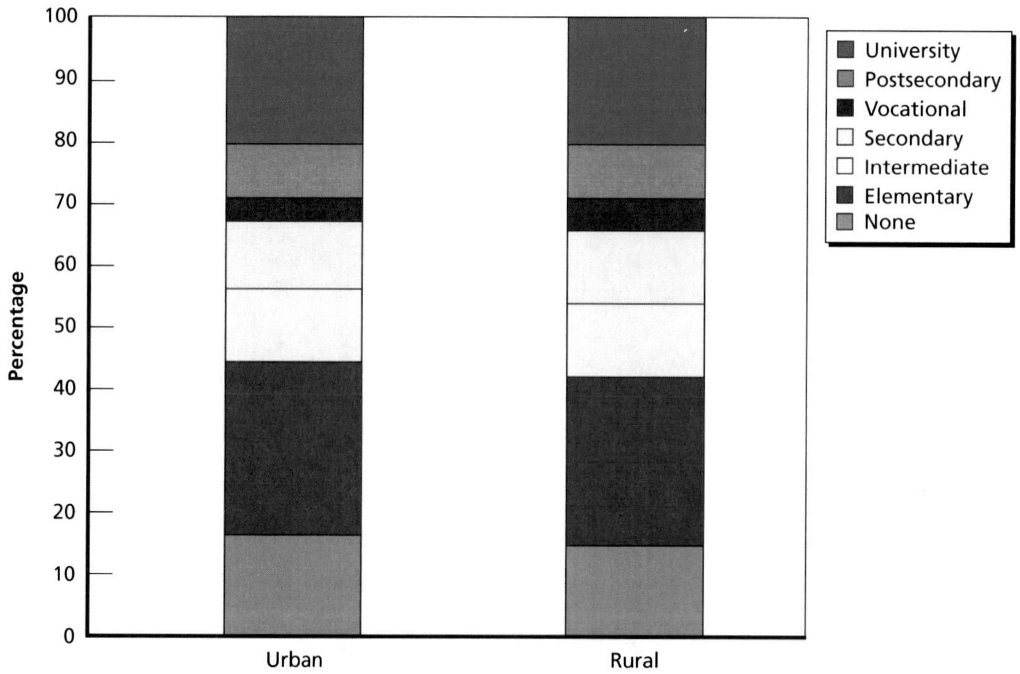

RAND *TR715-5.5*

Figure 5.6
Annual Household Spending on Education per Student (in dinars)

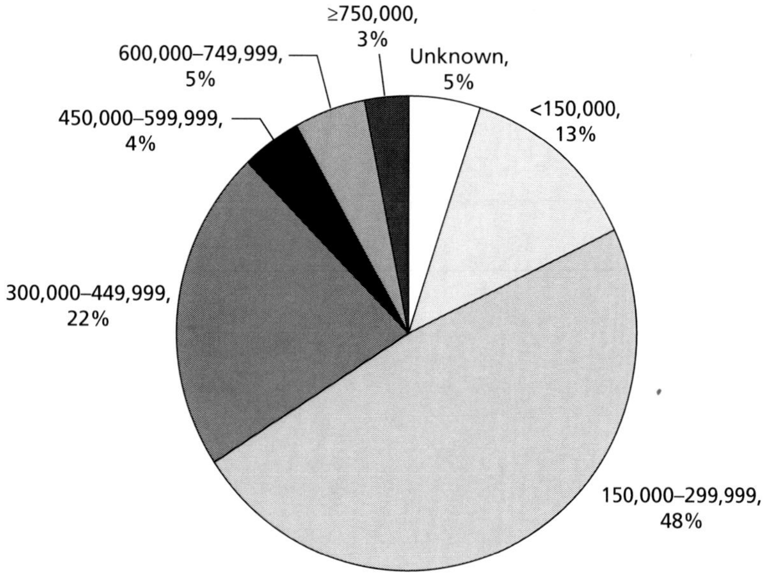

RAND *TR715-5.6*

Figure 5.7
Average Annual Cost of Education per Student, by Age

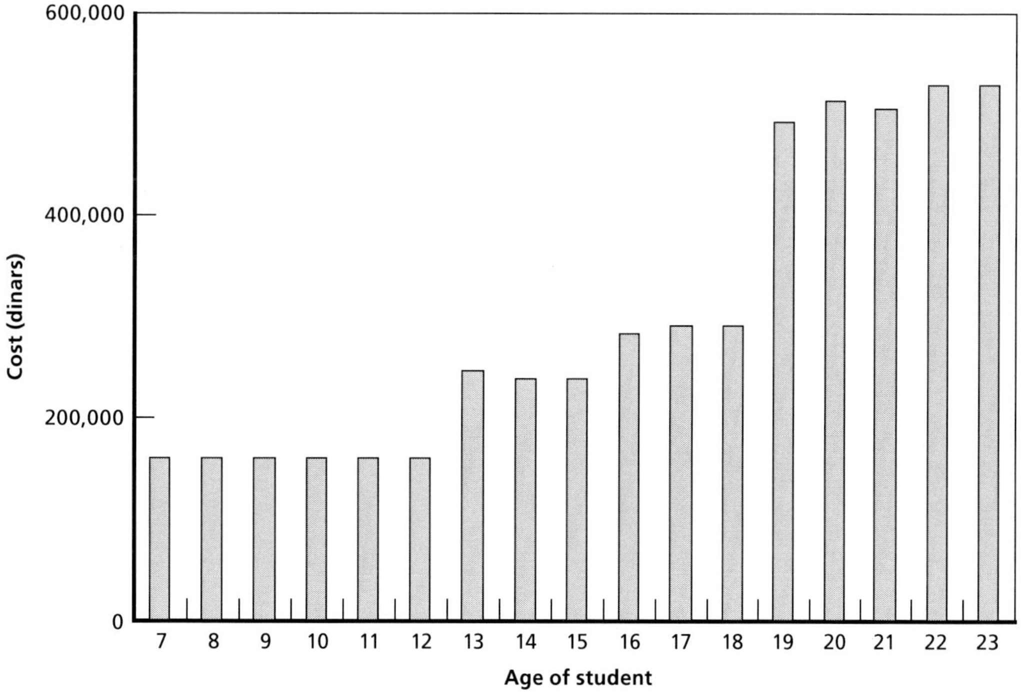

RAND *TR715-5.7*

between the elementary, intermediate, secondary, and university levels of education. Most of the money appears to be spent on tuition rather than uniforms, books, meals, or private lessons.[3] The amount spent on the latter group of expenses does not vary much by age.

---

[3] Costs are hardly uniform within any one age group. For instance, to educate 14-year-olds, 14 percent of all households spent an average of 150,000 dinars a year, 22 percent spent an average of 220,000 dinars, 33 percent spent an average of 250,000 dinars, and the rest spent an average of 300,000 dinars or more.

CHAPTER SIX

Health

Background

Health services in al-Anbar are provided by both the public and the private sectors. Major hospitals and clinics are government-owned and government-operated and are financed by the central government. Privately owned clinics and hospitals are usually smaller establishments that range from private doctor's clinics to small hospitals.

Drugs are not highly regulated in Iraq. Drug stores sell over the counter many drugs available only by prescription in the United States, including antibiotics. Anbari families' choices of forms of health care are determined by access to many medications without a prescription, traditions, the availability of trained professionals, accessibility, and the cost of obtaining health services (including the cost of transportation).

Survey Results

When ill, only 55 percent of respondents first turn to a trained health care professional (a category that includes nurses and midwives), as shown in Figure 6.1. Percentages are similar in both rural and urban areas.

Pharmacies are the largest single source of health care services. Most pharmacies in al-Anbar are small shops that get the bulk of their supplies from warehouses owned and operated by the Ministry of Health. Imported pharmaceuticals are significantly cheaper in Iraq than in neighboring countries because of government subsidies.

In many cases, drug stores are not operated by trained pharmacists. In some instances, employees are deemed adequately trained if they can read labels. Family members, not doctors or trained pharmacists, decide which medications to buy. As a result, antibiotics are often overused.

Both rural and urban households use traditional healers, midwives, and nurses. However, no respondents reported seeking medical treatment from religious leaders. As Figure 6.2 indicates, the likelihood that a household will seek health care from a professional appears to be independent of the level of education of the household head.

About 82 percent of household heads reported that primary health care is easily accessible. However, almost all respondents reported some or severe difficulty in seeing specialists, such as pediatricians, surgeons, or cardiologists. Most doctors, especially specialists, are located in urban centers. Patients travel to these centers for specialized treatment.

Figure 6.1
Source First Consulted for Health Care

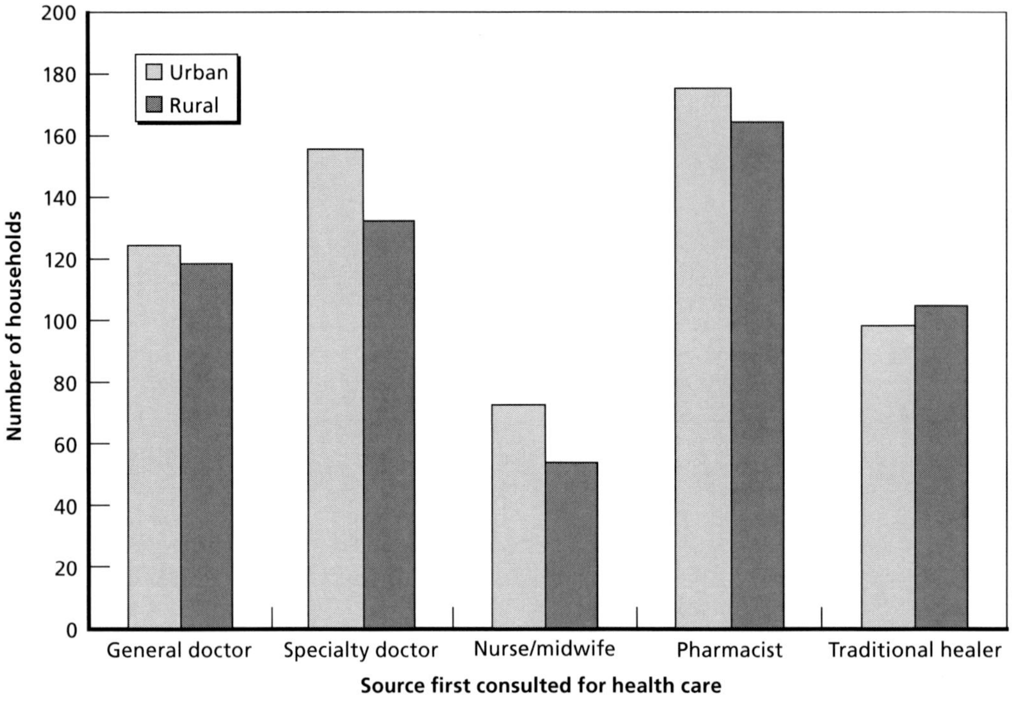

RAND *TR715-6.1*

Figure 6.2
Percentage of Households That Consult with Medical Professionals First, by Education Level of Household Head

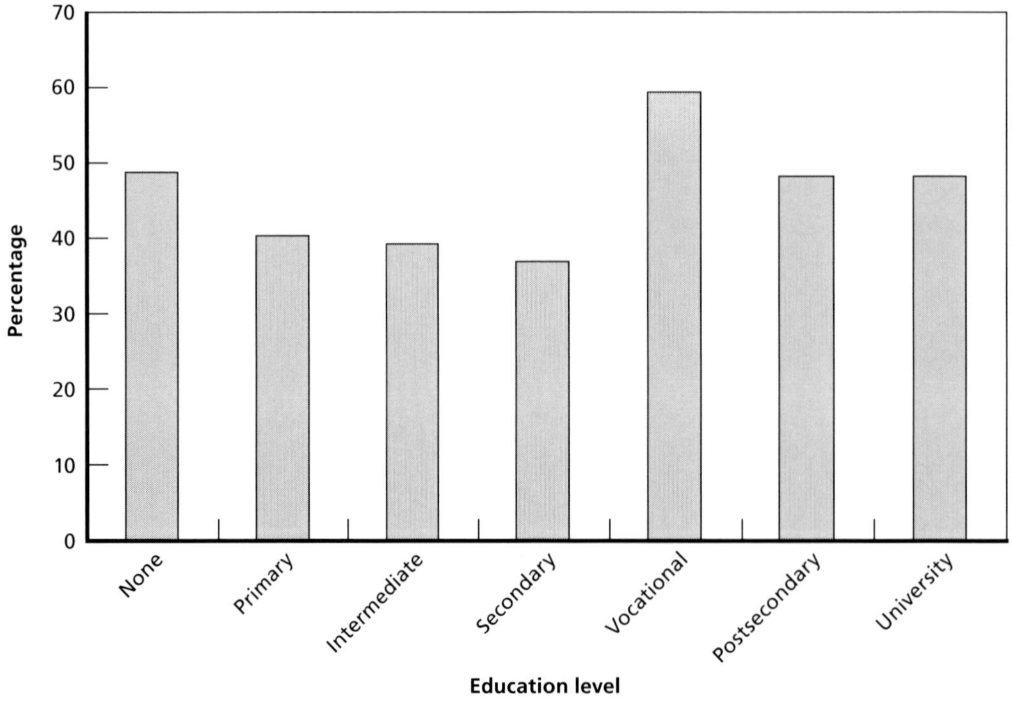

RAND *TR715-6.2*

Figure 6.3 shows that about one-quarter of those surveyed find it difficult to access government-sponsored clinics where vaccinations are available.[1] More than two-thirds of those surveyed report difficulties in getting emergency care, even though such care was government-provided. Dental care is slightly more accessible: Only 22 percent said it is difficult to obtain appointments with dentists.

Not surprisingly, it is harder to get appointments with caregivers who are more highly trained (see Figure 6.4). Midwives and nurses are relatively easy to see; specialist doctors are the hardest. Almost all respondents said that they have easy access to pharmacists.

Roughly 40 percent of those surveyed said they find it difficult to afford specialist care (see Figure 6.5). Although dental care is accessible, it is less affordable. As many health care professionals have fled the country, out-of-pocket health care costs have risen sharply, and both specialists and general practitioners often demand private payments. Because the Iraqi government covers most of the costs of emergency care, survey respondents find emergency care affordable.

Almost all survey respondents, rural and urban, live near a physician and a pharmacy. The median travel time is in the 15-minute range (see Figure 6.6, which combines average rural and urban travel times).[2] More importantly, no one lives so far from either a physician or pharmacist that he or she would be unable to access one or the other in a medical emergency. The cost of care and the ease of getting appointments, rather than travel time, appear to be the primary reasons why Anbaris turn to pharmacists for health care before seeking a doctor.

Figure 6.3
Ease of Access to Various Forms of Health Care

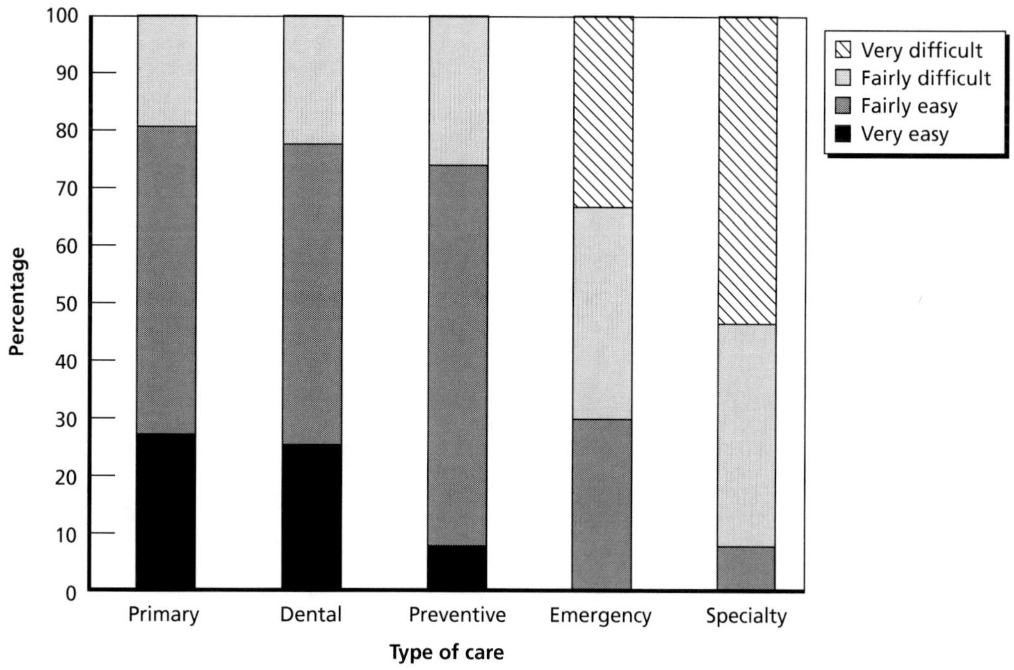

RAND *TR715-6.3*

---

[1] All vaccinations are government-provided and usually administered in hospitals or government-owned clinics. Private clinics rarely administer vaccinations.

[2] In 2004, 65 percent of Anbaris reported living within 15 minutes of a physician; the 2008 figure is 75 percent. Similarly, in 2004, 46 percent reported living within 15 minutes of a pharmacy; the 2008 figure is 61 percent.

Figure 6.4
Ease of Obtaining Appointments with Different Health Care Professionals

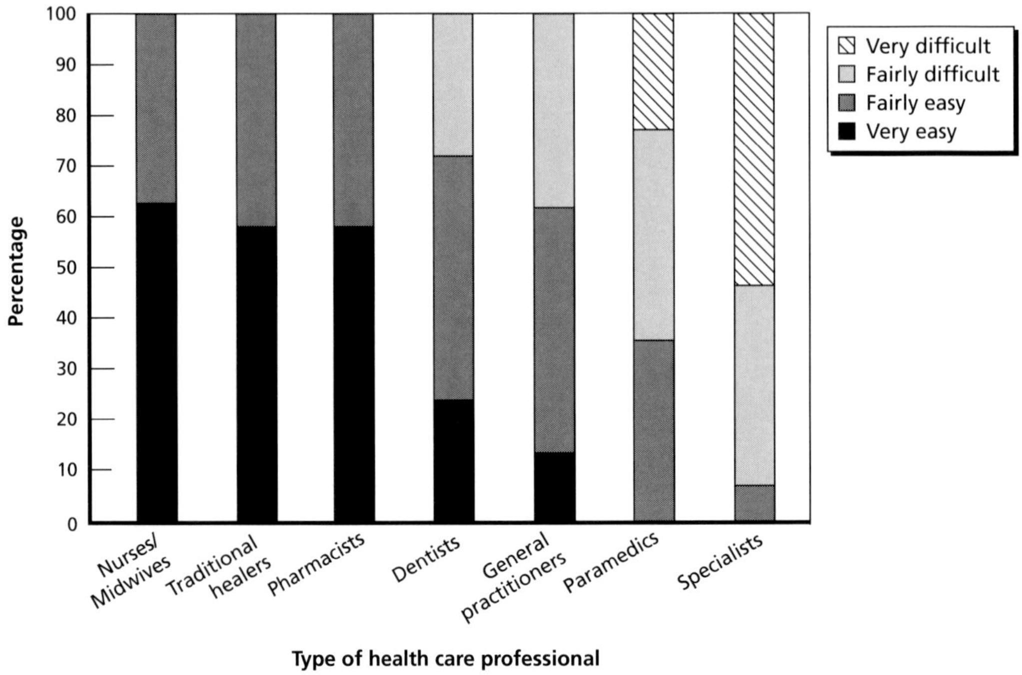

RAND *TR715-6.4*

Figure 6.5
Affordability of Health Care

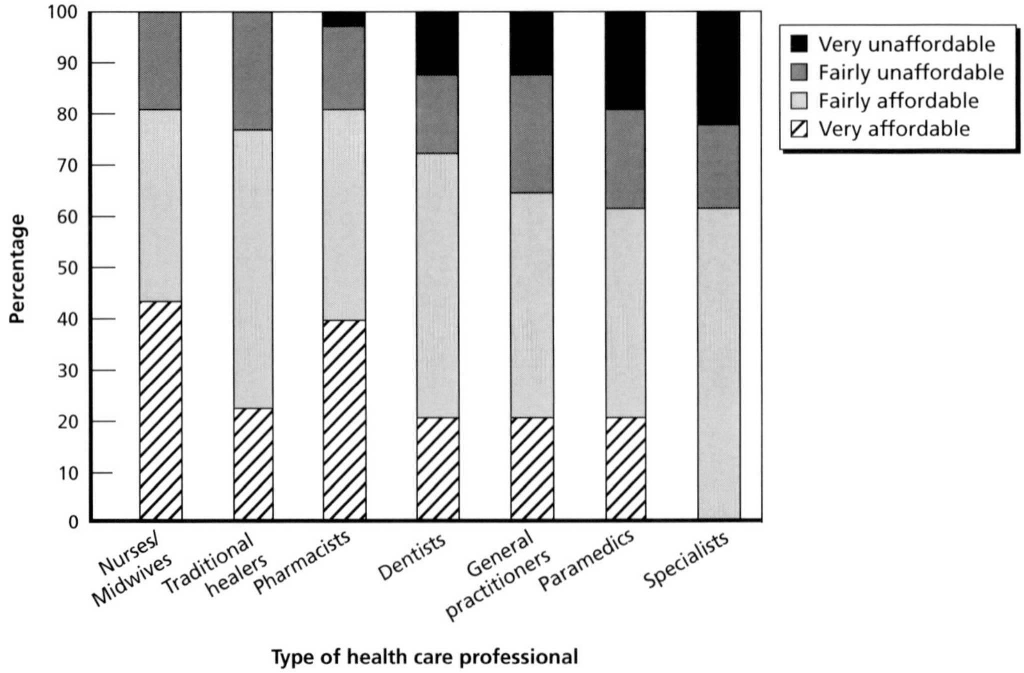

RAND *TR715-6.5*

Figure 6.6
Average Travel Time to Physicians and Pharmacies

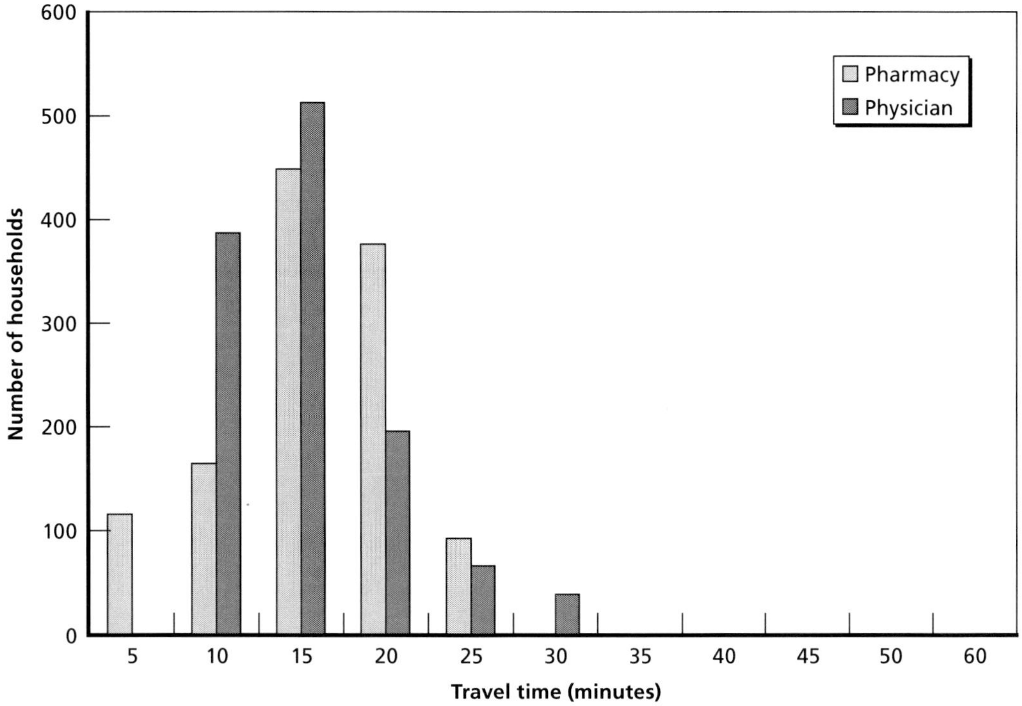

RAND *TR715-6.6*

Most of the respondents said that access to health care, notably access to nurses and midwives, has gotten easier since 2004 (see Figure 6.7). These answers are consistent across urban and rural population samples. However, it was more difficult in 2008 to get an appointment with a specialist or access emergency care compared with 2004.

In 2004, 13 percent of survey respondents said that the time required to travel to a physician was more than 30 minutes. In 2008, less than 5 percent of survey respondents said travel time to a physician was 30 minutes, and no one said it took more than 30 minutes to get to a doctor (see Figure 6.6).

The Iraqi government was the main provider of health care in 2004. In 2008, Anbaris were more likely to rely on foreign and local NGOs, such as the Red Crescent, for health care than on government-operated or privately operated facilities (see Figure 6.8).

Seventy percent of those surveyed use personal savings to pay for health care (see Figure 6.9). No one turns to such groups as international organizations, NGOs, tribes, political parties, or other local organizations to pay for medical care. Borrowing money from banks or credit institutions is also not an option. However, some are able to turn to the government. Religious organizations and community leaders also provide assistance at times. **None of the respondents indicated that outside groups, a category that could encompass violent groups, provide financial assistance for medical care.**

According to respondents, the four greatest problems with health care are, in order, the fact that a large number of health care professionals have left Iraq, the lack of health care supplies and equipment, the limited range of health services available nearby, and unsanitary facilities. A small number cited the distance to health care facilities as a problem (see Figure 6.10).

Figure 6.7
Ease of Obtaining Appointments with Various Health Care Workers (2008 compared with 2004)

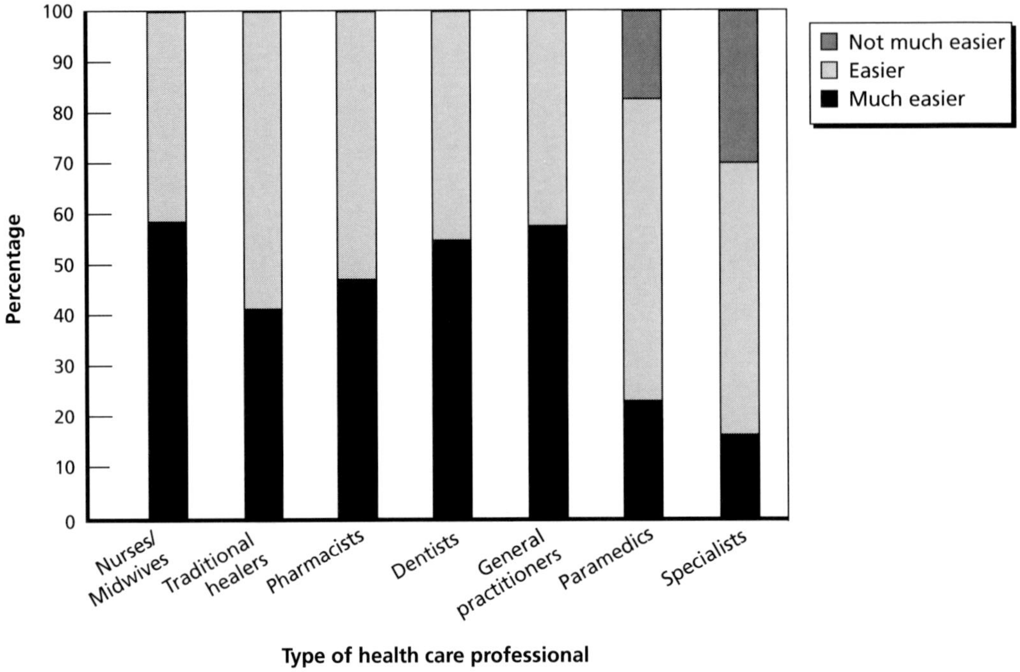

RAND *TR715-6.7*

Figure 6.8
Health Care Providers, by Institution Type

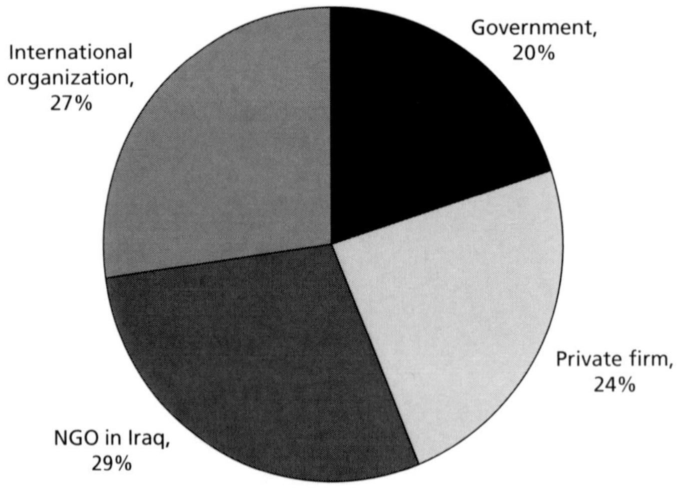

RAND *TR715-6.8*

Figure 6.9
Source of Health Care Financing

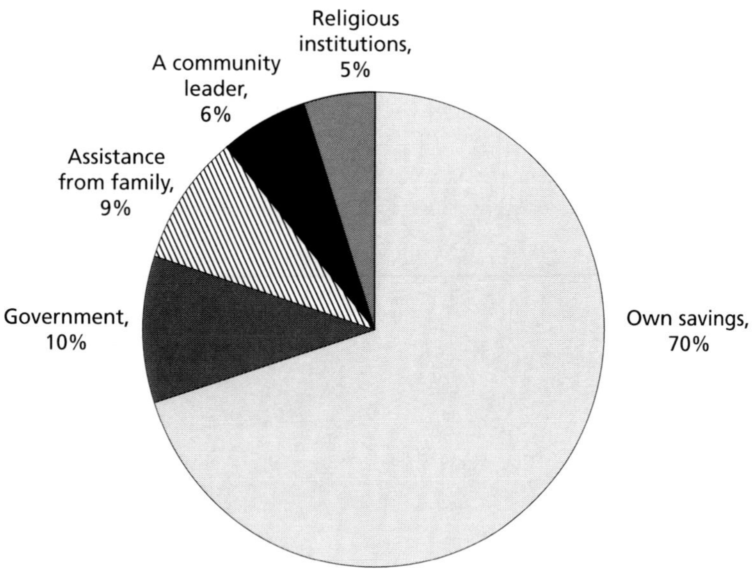

RAND *TR715-6.9*

Figure 6.10
Top Reported Problems in Iraq's Health Care System

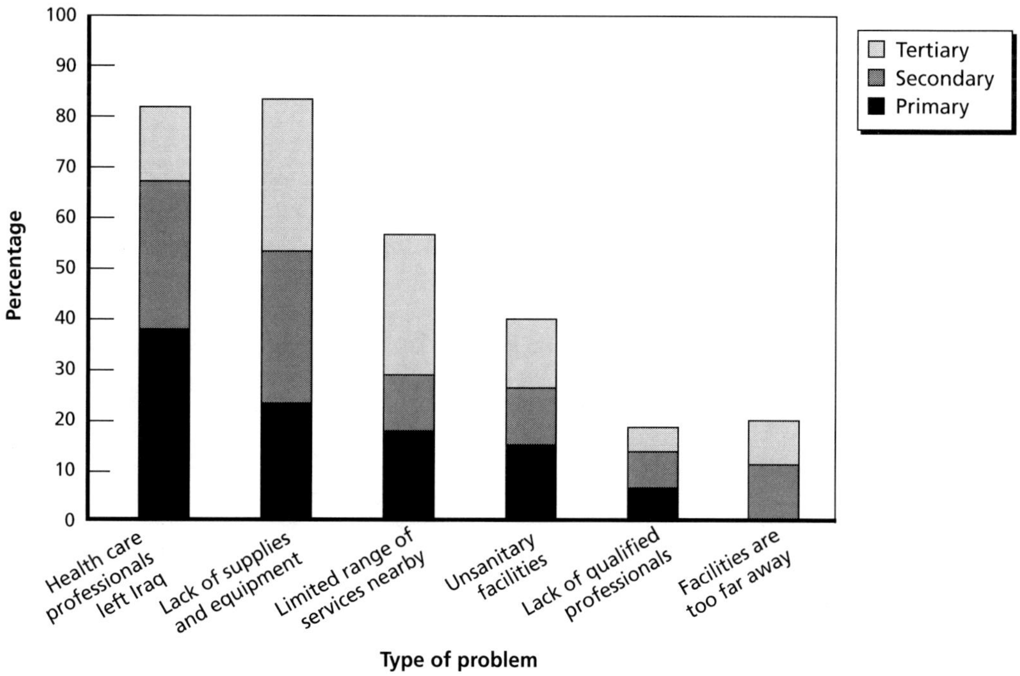

RAND *TR715-6.10*

CHAPTER SEVEN

Housing and Public Infrastructure

Background

Iraq's utilities and infrastructure are largely owned and operated by the Iraqi government. Because of its relatively favorable political position under Saddam Hussein, al-Anbar had enjoyed better service and better quality infrastructure than many other provinces (especially those in the south, where Shia are in the majority). However, both services and infrastructure seriously deteriorated in the 1990s because of damage from the first Gulf War, the decline in Iraq's budget revenues, United Nations sanctions, corruption (which siphoned off funds destined for public services and investment in infrastructure), and poor maintenance practices. Improvements in infrastructure were slowed by violence between 2003 and 2006, but since 2007, they have proceeded more quickly.

Survey Results

Anbari homes and apartments tend to be larger than those in countries with similar incomes, but the family sizes are smaller. More than 79 percent of respondents said their home contained five rooms or more. Most households use two or three rooms as bedrooms (see Figure 7.1); the remaining rooms are common rooms used by the entire family. Compared with most homes in the United States, Iraqi homes are crowded, with two or three people sleeping in each bedroom. This state of affairs has not changed since 2004: The report from the 2004 survey notes that "many families have to put up with crowded living conditions to stay in houses they can afford."[1]

Household size is weakly correlated with the number of rooms in a home (see Figure 7.2). Larger families do not necessarily have larger homes. As families get larger, households often become more crowded.

Among Anbari dwellings, 41 percent have garden plots, and 36 percent have a balcony. Anbari households that own or rent repair shops or workshops usually own or rent premises separately from their dwellings. Only 11 percent of houses are attached to a shop. Less than 3 percent of residences also house a workshop.

Almost 30 percent of all households rent out rooms. Income from rents averages 2.8 million dinars a year (roughly $2,300 a year or $192 a month). Rents are paid either in cash or

[1] Ministry of Planning and Development Cooperation, 2005. The Iraqi government also reported that 10 percent of Anbari households live in crowded conditions, which the UNDP defines as three or more persons per room. Using a slightly different criterion—more than four or more persons per bedroom—13 percent of Anbari households may be characterized as crowded.

Figure 7.1
Percentage of Anbari Households, by Number of Bedrooms in Dwelling

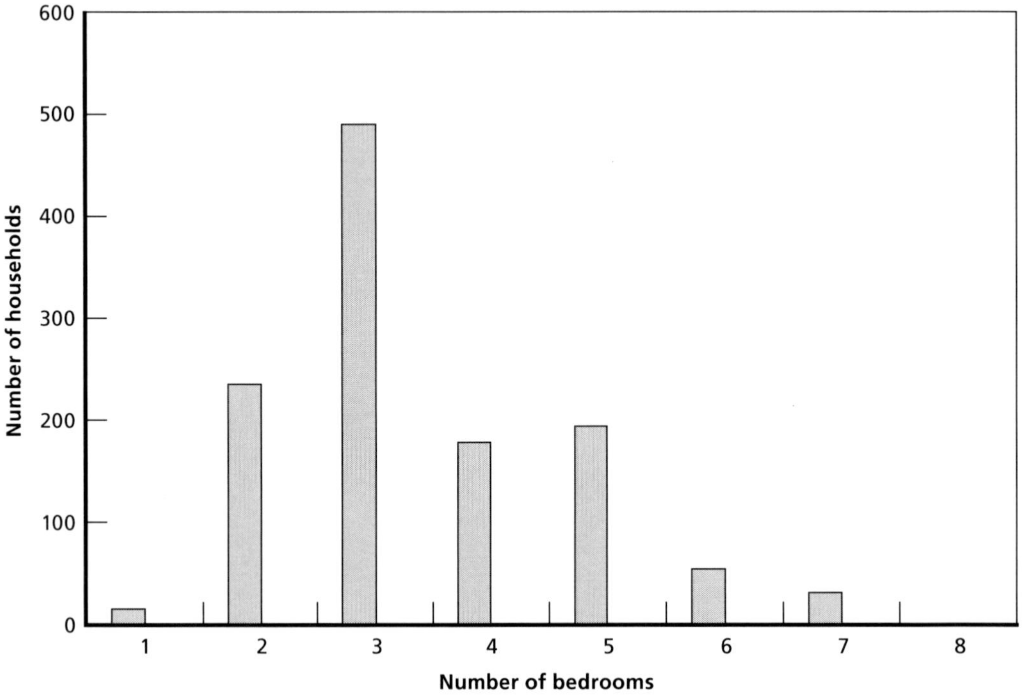

RAND *TR715-7.1*

Figure 7.2
Average Number of Bedrooms and Other Rooms

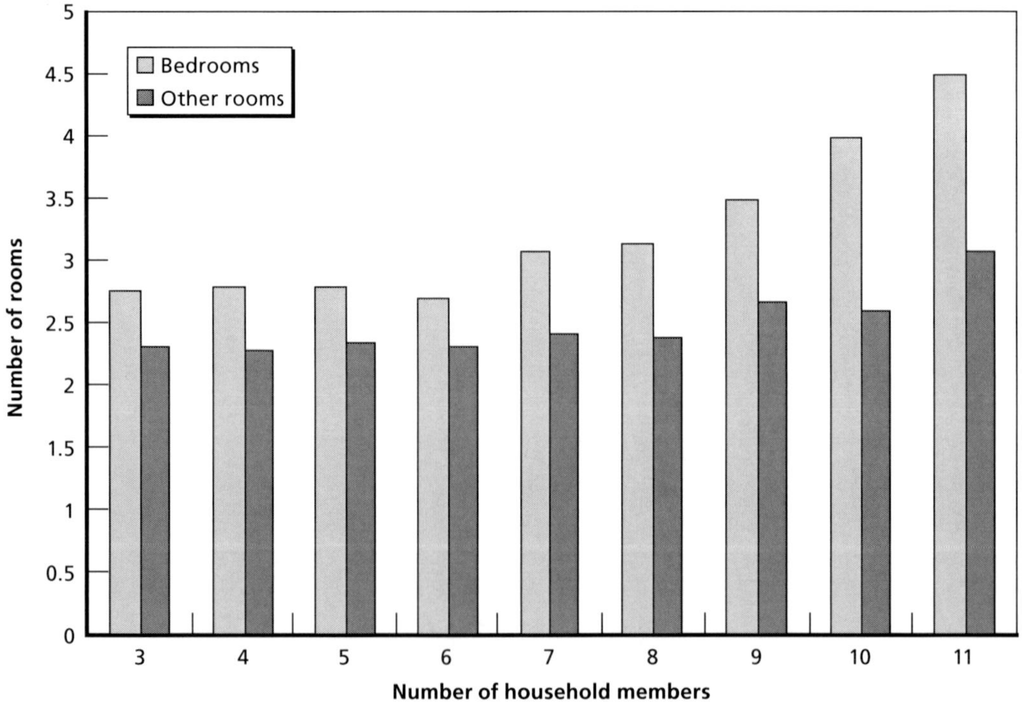

RAND *TR715-7.2*

in-kind (i.e., in exchange for food or services, such as repair services). In some instances, other members of the household pay rent, but in most instances, rents are earned by renting space to people other than household members.

Most households reported that their homes are in disrepair. The most frequently cited problem was lack of maintenance (52 percent). However, 11 percent reported damage due either to military activities (6.5 percent) or to a combination of lack of maintenance and military activities (4.5 percent). About a fourth (22 percent) of households said that at least one room in the home cannot be used because it has been heavily damaged. **Most households reported that they either have started repairing damage to their homes (22 percent) or have concrete plans to do so (44 percent). This repair activity is reflected in the resurgence in construction in al-Anbar.** Most households plan to conduct repairs using their own funds (41 percent) or money from their extended family (23 percent). Seven percent expect help from a community leader. Another 23 percent lack the funds to begin repairs.

Over the course of the last five years of conflict, many Anbari households have experienced extensive damage to their homes. The 2004 survey found that only 5 percent of homes in Iraq had experienced damage from military activity, and only 6 percent of households reported damage due to other factors, including lack of maintenance.

Every household reported using propane gas for cooking. In addition, 11.5 percent of households reported using kerosene, and 20.8 percent reported using electricity. No other fuels are used for cooking. All households use kerosene for heating. However, some also use small electric heaters (17 percent) or heaters that run on propane (5 percent). These figures are similar to those reported after the 2004 survey, which found that 87 percent of Iraqi households used kerosene to heat their homes. However, electricity is a more important secondary source of heating in al-Anbar than elsewhere in Iraq.

Al-Anbar continues to be plagued by electric power outages. **All the households rely on a diesel-powered generator (shared with neighbors, operated by a neighborhood cooperative, or run by a local private company) for electricity when electricity is not available from the grid.** As many as 30 percent of households have private generators, and 15 percent of households are connected to a private electric power network.

Most Anbari households reported that their electricity supply is unstable. All households reported some interruption in electricity supplies (see Figure 7.3). However, supply from the grid appears to have improved since 2004, when 81 percent of Anbar's population reported that their power supply was unstable (i.e., that they suffered prolonged daily blackouts).

Among surveyed households, 34 percent have access to the public sewage network, 57 percent use a septic tank, and the remainder use both. Eighty-four percent reported having a flush toilet connected to either a public sewage system or a septic tank. Anbari households also reported using outhouses. Judging by the United Nations standard for sanitation, which requires that household sewage systems be connected to public networks, al-Anbar's sanitation system can be characterized as being *improved* or *adequate*. However, Anbaris are unhappy with their sanitation systems. Up to 61 percent reported having frequent problems with the sewage network, and half reported that the sewage network never works properly.

The majority of households (60 percent) dispose of trash by dumping it themselves, but not in a publicly designated landfill. Roughly 15 percent use other means to get rid of garbage, notably burning. Fewer than 10 percent enjoyed regular garbage collection.

All households surveyed reported piped-in water as their main source of water. A minority of households rely on tanker-truck vendors (11 percent) and covered public wells (8 per-

Figure 7.3
Consistency of Electric Power Supply

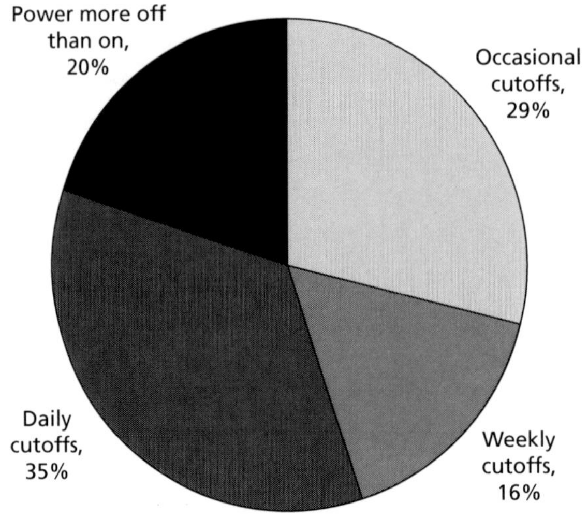

RAND *TR715-7.3*

cent) to augment supplies. Every household graded its water supply as reliable, but 39 percent reported occasional but less-often-than-weekly problems, 35 percent reported weekly problems, and 27 percent reported daily problems. Just over half of all households strongly disagreed with the statement that their household "has no problem obtaining the drinking water . . . [it] need[s]."

There appears to be little systematic difference between urban and rural households in matters such as electricity supply and travel time, although there are differences when it comes to water and sewage issues. All urban households are connected to public sewage lines, but only a quarter of rural households are connected; conversely, all rural households have septic tanks, but only 70 percent of urban households do. Twenty percent of urban households discard their trash in open public containers, but no rural residents do. Finally, no urban head of households strongly disagrees with the proposition that his or her household always has an adequate supply of water, but almost 30 percent of rural head of household take serious issue with such a characterization.

These figures largely correspond with the 2004 survey, which found that 88 percent of all urban households in Iraq use piped-in water as their main source of drinking water. In addition, that survey reported that 33 percent of all Iraqi households have an unstable supply of drinking water.

Ease of travel to public facilities varies by type of facility, as shown in Figure 7.4. Over 90 percent of Anbaris can get to their closest mosque within 15 minutes. However, only 20 percent can get to their closest police station within 20 minutes. Anbari households claim to have relatively easy access to various educational and medical facilities. As many as 84 percent live within 15 minutes of an elementary school, and 86 percent live within 25 minutes of a secondary school.

Of the Anbari households surveyed, more than half (54 percent) use their own cars. Most of the rest (34 percent) use a taxi, and the remainder use public transportation.

Figure 7.4
Travel Time to Various Destinations

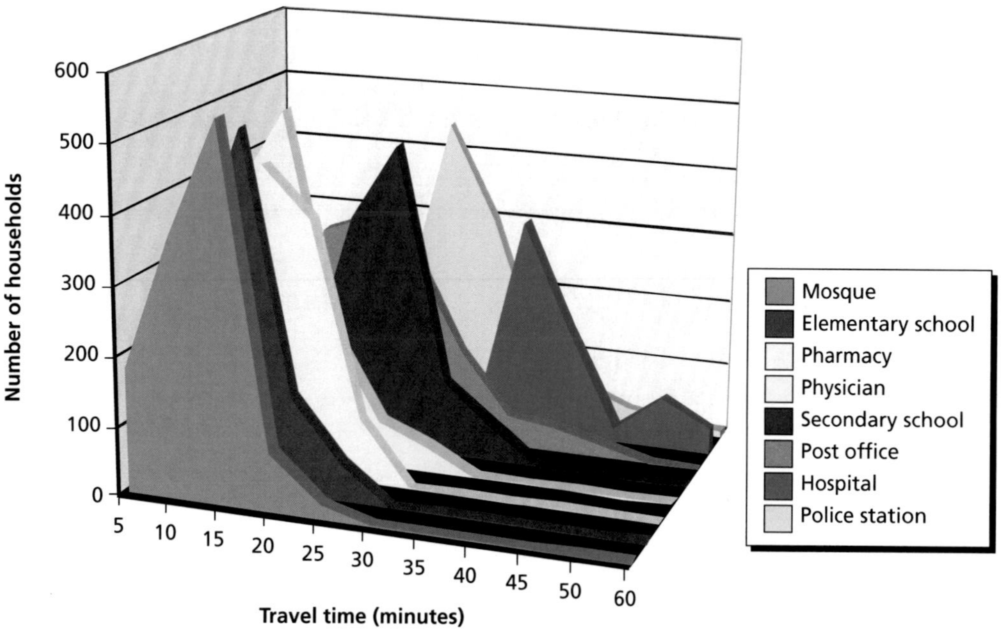

RAND *TR715-7.4*

CHAPTER EIGHT

The Effects of War

Background

As the center of AQI's activity in 2006 and the most prominent part of the deadly "Sunni Triangle" following the U.S. invasion in 2003, al-Anbar was once the most violent province in Iraq. Violence fell sharply in 2007 and has continued to abate. Al-Anbar is now enjoying its lowest levels of violence since 2003, with especially dramatic declines in Fallujah and Ramadi.

Survey Results

Deaths, Injury, Displacement, and Crime

The 2008 survey found that 47 percent of households surveyed claimed that at least one household member had been killed between spring 2006 and spring 2008. As shown in Figure 8.1, approximately 36 percent reported that a household member had gone missing, and 11 percent reported that a household member had been forced to flee or had otherwise been displaced. Coupled with reporting on damage to homes and numbers of widows and fatherless children, this survey shows very high levels of suffering from conflict in al-Anbar. In addition to the consequences of war, levels of crime are high: 9 percent of households reported that someone in their household had been a victim of crime within the last four weeks.

An examination of the distribution across al-Anbar of households that have experienced the effects of war shows that the various parts of the province report similar trends. For example,

- In Ramadi, 51 percent of households surveyed reported that at least one household member had been killed due to war-related violence. In Fallujah, 46 percent reported the same.
- In Ramadi, 27 percent of households reported that a household member had been detained or arrested. In Fallujah, 23 percent reported the same.

Relocation

Eighteen percent of the households surveyed reported that at least one member had relocated out of al-Anbar since 2003. Such members had usually left sometime between 2004 and 2006. Violence was the main reason cited for leaving. The need to search for work or to leave home to attend school or university were other frequently cited, more-benign reasons for leaving.

Figure 8.1
Percentage of Households That Have Felt Specific Effects of War and Crime

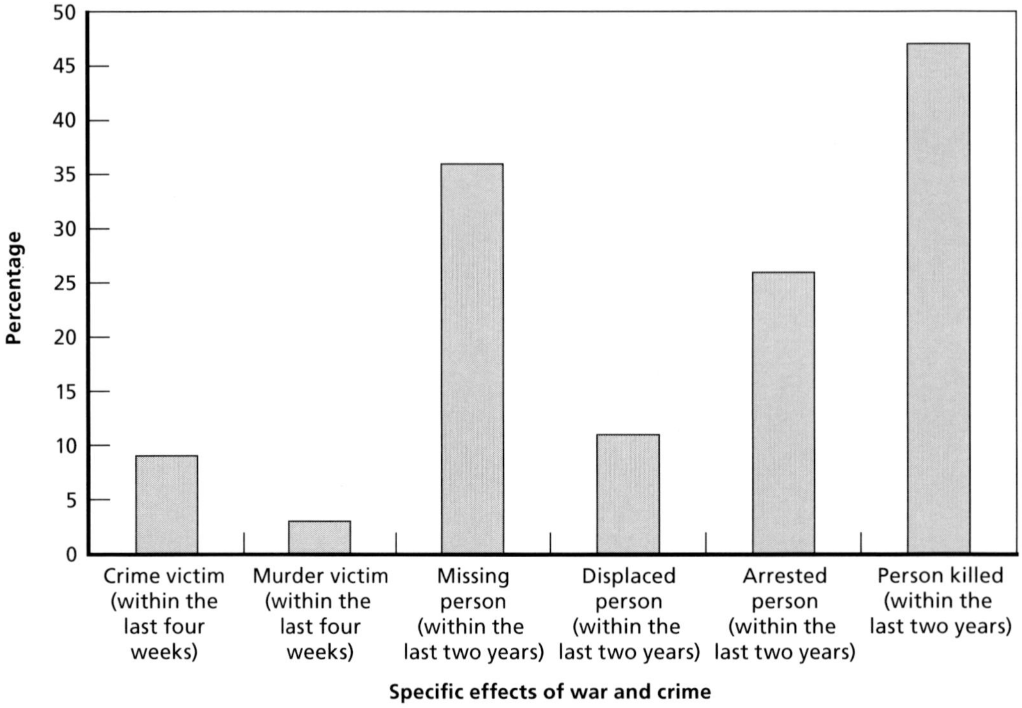

As shown in Figure 8.2, roughly half of survey respondents said that the household member who left migrated to Syria (59 percent); other foreign destinations were Jordan (12 percent), Egypt (8 percent), and Sweden (6 percent). Comparatively fewer (15 percent) relocated internally in Iraq, but those who did moved to areas further north, including Kurdistan (10 percent) and the predominantly Sunni Arab Salah-ad-din (5 percent).

The closer the household lives to Syria, the more likely it is that the departing member relocated there. Table 8.1 shows both the number of departing Anbaris as a ratio of total residents (by area within al-Anbar) and the percentage of those who moved to Syria.

Displacement patterns in Ramadi and Fallujah are similar: 18 percent and 16 percent, respectively, of households in these two cities reported that a household member had relocated elsewhere. About as many left alone (56 percent) as left with other household members (44 percent). More of the individuals who left Ramadi had worked in the public sector (35 percent) than in the private sector (21 percent).

From urban Fallujah, 63 percent left alone rather than with other household members (37 percent). As in Ramadi, violence was the main reason cited for leaving, although roughly 10 percent left to look for work and another 10 percent left to go to school.

Displacement in rural households in al-Anbar (18 percent) is on par with the urban rate. The most significant years of migration were 2004 and 2005. Individual household members in rural regions were essentially just as likely to depart their homes alone (52 percent) as to leave with other household members (48 percent). As in the urban regions, fully 60 percent of individuals left due to violent conditions; roughly a tenth left for school-related reasons, and about 8 percent left for work-related reasons.

Figure 8.2
Where Emigrating Anbaris Go

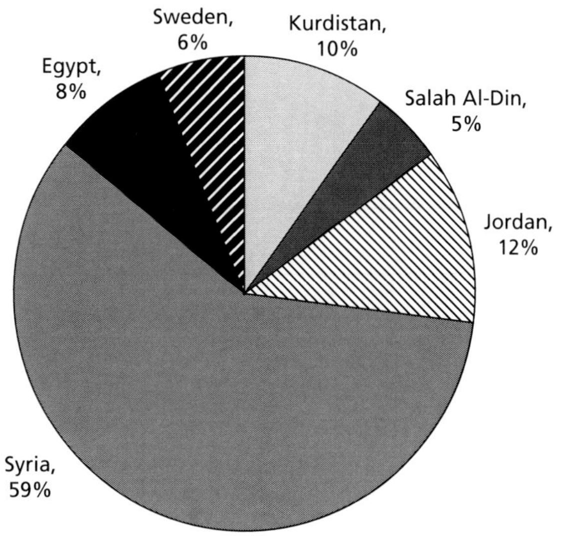

RAND *TR715-8.2*

Table 8.1
Relocation, by Region

Area Within al-Anbar	Survey Population	Departures	Ratio of Departures to Survey Population	Percentage of Departees Who Moved to Syria
West	2,417	91	0.038	78
Center	2,941	102	0.035	66
East	2,843	110	0.039	52

New Residents

Anbari households, as opposed to individual members of the households, have not moved much. The vast majority of households (94 percent) said that they had lived in their current residence since 2005 or before. Just 6 percent of households had moved into their current residence since 2005. **When those who had moved were asked why they had done so, the largest group answered that the area they moved from had not been secure.** Most of the new arrivals came from Baghdad (see Figure 8.3). The rate of movement within al-Anbar was much lower.

Figure 8.3
Where New Arrivals to al-Anbar Come From

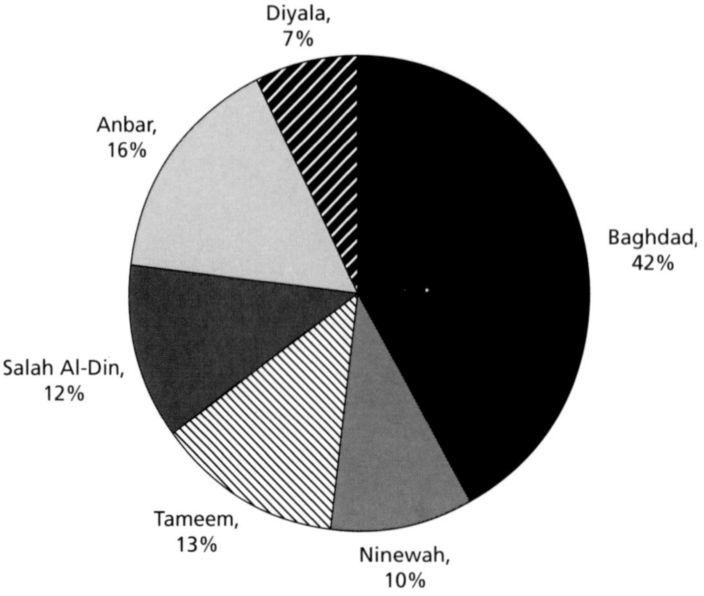

RAND *TR715-8.3*

CHAPTER NINE

Agriculture

Background

According to the 2004 survey, agriculture was the third-largest field of employment in Iraq: 17 percent of the entire Iraqi labor force was employed in agriculture. Only trade and government were larger employment sectors. Because the Euphrates runs through al-Anbar, the province is agriculturally productive. Moreover, it does not suffer as much from the problems of salinization that plague the south.

Agricultural equipment, seeds, pesticides, and fertilizers have been heavily subsidized in Iraq. The government has also guaranteed purchases and prices for specific crops while imposing hefty tariffs to keep out competing products from other countries. Tariffs have been reduced and input subsidies cut since 2004 to provide incentives for Iraqi farmers to grow the crops that Iraqi households desire and to operate more efficiently.

Survey Results

Land Ownership

As Figure 9.1 shows, almost one in three households in al-Anbar owns land, and two out of five cultivate land. There is a strong correlation between land ownership and land cultivation. Among those households who own land, 53 percent cultivate; among those who do not own land, only 17 percent cultivate.

Roughly 19 percent of the households surveyed rent land from others. Many rent from relatives, some of whom have left Iraq. Others rent from local leaders. Historically, sheiks often owed their position to land holdings. The cost of renting arable land seems to be fairly constant across the province, averaging 650,000 dinars per *dunum*[1] (roughly $1,000/acre), with a high of 900,000 dinars ($1,400/acre) and a low of 450,000 dinars ($700/acre).

Because arable areas in al-Anbar are densely populated, and because most households, urban and rural, supplement their diets with food they produce themselves, both urban and rural dwellers report that they grow crops and own livestock (poultry—usually chickens—goats, and sheep). Dense population tends to keep holdings small: Over a third of all holdings in al-Anbar are 3 *dunum* (2 acres) or less. With holdings being small, few Anbaris make a living from farming alone: Only 4 percent of heads of household classified themselves as farmers.

[1] One *dunum* is equal to 0.618 acres.

Figure 9.1
Percentage of Households That Own or Cultivate Land

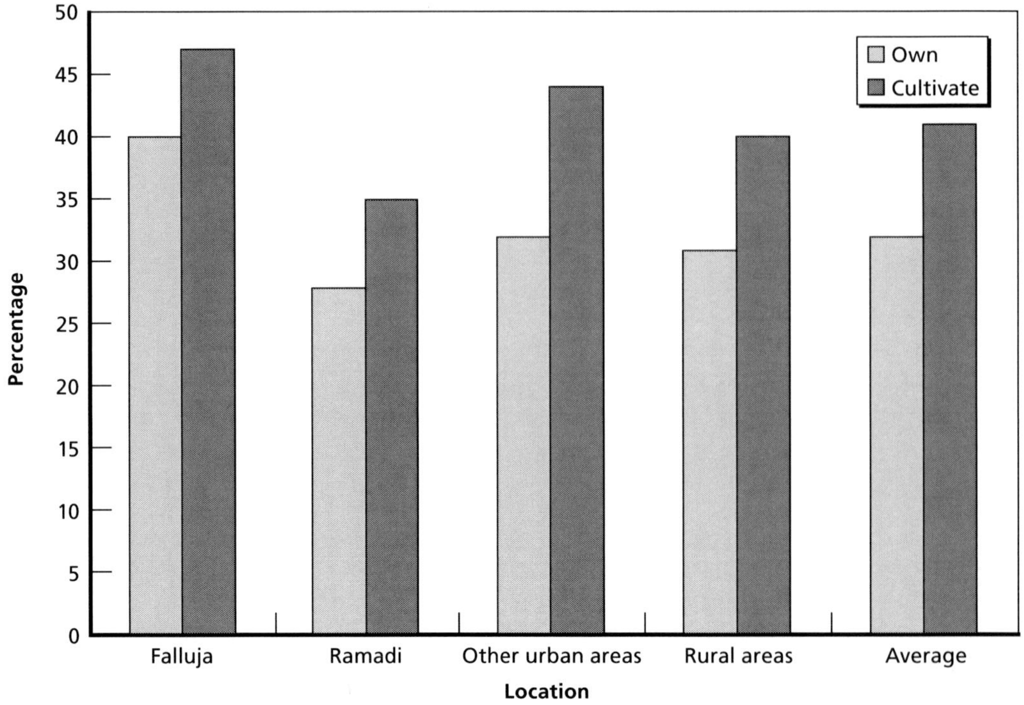

RAND *TR715-9.1*

Irrigation and Mechanization

Most farmers are able to irrigate part (but not all) of their farms. Two-fifths of farmers in rural areas said they do not have enough water to irrigate all the land that they wished to cultivate. Despite their wish to irrigate more land, their irrigation methods tend to be wasteful. Almost 40 percent of the irrigated land is watered by sprinklers or flooding. Iraqi farmers use the more parsimonious drip method on less than 10 percent of the land they cultivate. Because farmers do not pay for water, they have less incentive to use it more efficiently. More than three-quarters of farmers use pumps to irrigate their fields. In most instances, these pumps are motorized, but in some cases, they are powered by hand or by livestock.

Despite their small size, farms in al-Anbar tend to be mechanized: Two-thirds of Anbaris who farm use tractors and mechanical harvesters; about one-third use plows pulled by draft animals. However, much of the mechanized equipment is quite old and was purchased (and in some cases imported) used.

Almost half of the respondents own livestock. Goats and sheep are raised even in such urban areas as Ramadi and Fallujah. In keeping with the small scale of most farms, holdings of livestock are modest. Most owners reported anywhere between 7 and 25 livestock animals in almost all areas of al-Anbar. As levels of violence fell and economic activity increased between 2007 and 2008, holdings of livestock and poultry rose.

Bibliography

Al-Nasrawi, Abbas, "Economic Consequences of the Iraq-Iran War," *Third World Quarterly*, Vol. 8, No. 3, July 1986.

Al-Zabir, Mawiya, "Ni'ām al-Ba'ath wa Ijtithāthihi wa Hijrat al-'Uqūl al-'Iraqiyya [The Ba'ath Regime and Its Uprooting and the Iraqi Brain Drain]," al-Jazeera.net, March 11, 2004. As of October 14, 2008: http://www.aljazeera.net/News/archive/archive?ArchiveId=72723

"Iraq: Anbar Province Plagued by Violence," *IRIN*, January 15, 2007. As of September 17, 2008: http://www.irinnews.org/Report.aspx?ReportId=64374

Asquith, Christina, "Iraq's Students Say, 'Welcome Back Professor,'" *Christian Science Monitor*, December 9, 2003.

Baram, Amatzia, "The Effect of Iraqi Sanctions: Statistical Pitfalls and Responsibility," *Middle East Journal*, Vol. 54, No. 2, Spring 2000.

Blacker, John, Gareth Jones, and Mohamed M. Ali, "Annual Mortality Rates and Excess Deaths of Children Under Five in Iraq, 1991–1998," *Population Studies,* Vol. 57, No. 2, 2003.

Cordesman, Anthony H., "The Iraq War: Key Trends and Developments," briefing, Center for Strategic International Studies, May 7, 2008.

Garfield, Richard, and Ron Waldman, "Review of Potential Interventions to Reduce Child Mortality in Iraq," paper, November 5, 2003.

International Crisis Group, "Iraq After the Surge I: The New Sunni Landscape," *Middle East Report No. 74*, April 30, 2008.

International Monetary Fund, *Iraq: Second Review Under the Stand-By Arrangement and Financing Assurances Review—Staff Report*, IMF Country Report No. 08/383, Washington, D.C., 2008.

"Iraq, Education, and Children of Conflict," transcript of an April 8, 2008 conference at the Council on Foreign Relations, Federal News Service, Inc., 2008. As of September 25, 2008: http://www.cfr.org/publication/15977/iraq_education_and_children_of_conflict_rush_transcript_federal_news_service.html

Jones, Seth G., Lee H. Hilborne, C. Ross Anthony, Lois M. Davis, Federico Girosi, Cheryl Benard, Rachel M. Swanger, Anita Datar Garten, and Anga R. Timilsina, *Securing Health: Lessons from Nation-Building Missions*, Santa Monica, Calif.: RAND Corporation, MG-321-RC, 2006. As of June 9, 2009: http://www.rand.org/pubs/monographs/MG321/

Marr, Phebe, *The Modern History of Iraq*, Boulder, Colo.: Westview Press, 2004.

Ministry of Planning and Development Cooperation, *Iraq Living Conditions Survey 2004*, Vol. II: *Analytical Report*, Baghdad: Central Organization for Statistics and Information Technology, Ministry of Planning and Development Cooperation, 2005.

O'Hanlon, Michael E., and Jason H. Campbell, "Iraq Index: Tracking Variables of Reconstruction & Security in Post-Saddam Iraq," Brookings Institution, April 24, 2008. As of September 24, 2008: http://www.brookings.edu/saban/iraq-index.aspx

Raghavan, Sudarsan, "A New Breed Grabs Reins in Anbar," *Washington Post*, October 22, 2008.

Special Inspector General for Iraq Reconstruction, *Quarterly Report and Semiannual Report*, April 30, 2008.

Tavernise, Sabrina, "Amid Iraqi Chaos, Schools Fill After Long Decline," *New York Times*, June 26, 2006.

United Nations Educational, Scientific and Cultural Organization Institute for Statistics, "Data Centre," Web page, undated. As of October 2008:
http://stats.uis.unesco.org/unesco/TableViewer/document.aspx?ReportId=143&IF_Language=eng

United Nations Statistics Division, "Millennium Development Goals Indicators: The Official United Nations Site for the MDG Indicators," Web page, undated. As of October 2008:
http://mdgs.un.org/unsd/mdg/Data.aspx

World Bank, "Country Brief: Middle East & North Africa (MENA)—Iraq," August 2006. As of October 2008:
http://siteresources.worldbank.org/INTIRAQ/Resources/IRAQ-ENG-2006AM.pdf

———, "Iraq," Web page, 2009. As of October 2008:
http://go.worldbank.org/VKTOEKWV50

World Health Organization, *The World Health Report—Make Every Mother and Child Count*, Geneva: World Health Organization, 2005, Statistical Annex. As of September 2008:
http://www.who.int/whr/2005/annexes-en.pdf